Healthcare Computing

A Guide to Health Information Management and Systems

by

Tim Benson

and

Roderick Neame

Healthcare Computing

Published by Longman Information & Reference
Longman Group Limited, Westgate House, The High,
Harlow, Essex CM20 1YR, United Kingdom.
Telephone: (0279) 442601
Facsimile: (0279) 444501

First Published 1994

© Longman Group Limited 1994

ISBN 0-582-22978-2

A catalogue record for this book is available from the British Library.

Printed in Great Britain by BPC Wheatons Ltd, Exeter

HEALTHCARE COMPUTING

Contents

About the authors

Tim Benson is Chairman of Abies Medical Information Systems Ltd. He founded Abies in 1980 to develop and market clinical information systems that help doctors and managers in their daily work. Abies' computer-based patient record systems cover more than 20 clinical specialties and most hospital activities.

During the 1980s Tim worked closely with James Read to develop the Read Codes. He has been committed to the development of standards for medical data interchange since 1987 and is covenor of the group responsible for developing standard healthcare messages and communications in Europe (CEN TC251 WG3). He has served as Chairman of the Computing Services Association's Healthcare Group and is a member of the Audit Commission's advisory group on information systems in acute hospitals. He has particular interests in doctor-computer interaction, standards, electronic data interchange, coding and classification, and outcome measures.

Prior to founding Abies, he led the computer evaluation team at the Charing Cross Hospital for six years, where he also worked on healthcare outcome measures with Rachel Rosser. He originally trained as an engineer and has a BSc and MSc from Nottingham University and a BA from the Open University. He has written a previous book "Medical Informatics" also published by Longman.

Timothy J R Benson BSc, MSc, BA (Open), Chairman, *Abies Medical Information Systems Ltd*, Abies House, 103 Barretts Green Road, London NW10 7AP, Tel: 081–961 9777, Fax: 081–961 7666.

Roddy Neame has extensive experience in the health sector as an academic teacher and researcher, as a director of information services and as a management consultant.

After completing his higher degree studies in England, Roddy emigrated to Australia in the late 1970s to help set up the educationally innovative medical school in Newcastle, New South Wales. This development is now recognised as a world leader in community-oriented, problem-based and integrated medical education.

He made his home in Newcastle for about 17 years, during which time he established the first department of medical informatics in Australia, played a leading role in setting up the professional association for health informatics in NSW, chaired the committee for health informatics standards for Australia and New Zealand, and acted as area director for medical informatics for the Hunter region of NSW. He now lives with his wife and 4 children in Kent.

He has spent much of the past 20 years as a consultant with clients mainly in the Middle and Far East, and in Australasia. He was director of the assistance project to help establish the new medical school in Bahrain. Recently he has helped develop the national health information network for the Ministry of Health in New Zealand. He has run numerous courses in health informatics and has published more than 100 articles on health informatics, human physiology, medical education and clinical reasoning. He has special interests in health information, communication and networks, privacy and security, education, training and management of change, and smart cards.

Dr Roderick L B Neame MA, MB, BChir (Cantab), PhD (Lond) is chief executive of *Health Informatics Consulting*, Homestall, Kent ME13 8UT, England. Tel: 0795 539996, Fax: 0795 538390.

Foreword

Everyone who works in the health service will feel impact of information technology over the next few years. In the new health service it is vital to please purchasers, and information is all that most purchasers actually see for their money. Quality information has become essential for securing the income, and survival, of each provider unit.

The volume of information generated in the health service is massive. Each year the NHS generates over one billion forms, most of which stand to be replaced by computer-generated messages. The growth of information systems is inevitable.

Yet, the implementation of healthcare computing has proven far slower and more difficult than anyone imagined. Even today there is not a single hospital, anywhere in the world, where the computer systems meet the full expectations of all doctors, nurses and managers.

The prime aim of this book is to educate healthcare staff about what really matters in healthcare computing and information management. We have set out to provide core knowledge of the key topics and issues which separate success from failure. The emphasis is on presenting the most important principles and on how to realise the benefits which can be achieved.

Do not try to read it from start to finish. Use the contents page and the index to find the parts of greatest interest to you.

We hope that this book helps you obtain and use systems that meet your needs and expectations.

Chapter 1 The opportunity

Overview

Healthcare is an information intensive service industry. Vast amounts of information are generated and stored in hospitals, GP surgeries, community health services, clinical laboratories and in the many other healthcare services. Perhaps one third of all staff time is devoted to information processing tasks which could be computerised. However, most healthcare information is still handled using methods which have been little influenced by advances in technology, often making it difficult to retrieve the information for reuse or analysis, and leading to frequent duplication of care services as a consequence.

World-wide, healthcare systems are reeling under the burden of runaway costs. More and more can be done to keep people alive and well for longer, but this costs money. The rising costs of care, together with escalating patient expectations are combining to put pressure on budgets.

Many governments have responded to this challenge by:

- Capping expenditure, resulting in growing waiting lists
- Restricting availability of services to certain population groups, resulting in growing inequity of access

These do little to resolve the real problem. In the longer term we have to improve the effectiveness and efficiency with which services are selected and delivered, and reduce the risks of premature death and avoidable illness. However, attempts to implement and assess risk reduction strategies are hampered by the lack of essential information.

Health sector reforms designed to increase the competition between provider units may make some contribution. However, the greatest contribution will come from the appropriate use of computers and information technology. This will achieve major benefits in terms of:

- **Cost savings** — by automating manual information processing procedures
- **Quality of care** — by providing fast and reliable access to information

1

- **Improved service delivery** — by using trustworthy and relevant management information

Optimum use of information management and technology should deliver as much as a 40 per cent economy.

Future directions

The next decade or two will bring radical changes, many of which will be dependent upon information systems for their viability. The driving force behind these changes must be financial in the final analysis — without a sound basis of self-interest and profit no development, however desirable, has any real chance of success. Many of the imperatives will arise out of political and philosophical considerations. Appropriate manipulation of the incentive and reward structures in the care system can convert these into financial imperatives.

The way most of us access healthcare advice and expertise will also change markedly. Less healthcare delivery will take place within hospitals and existing care facilities. Services will be more focused on patient convenience and wishes, and will be delivered using networks that extend to homes and local community centres.

The following are some of the developments that we will be seeing in the near future. Some have already started to happen, whilst others are not quite there yet. They have been assembled into four groups for the purposes of this discussion:

- The provision of information
- Movement of information
- Infrastructure developments
- Virtual environments

Provision of information

Administrative support

The complex administrative requirements of the healthcare system will be extensively automated. Statistical information from operational healthcare systems will be immediately accessible to administrators at all levels for analysis and review using executive information management tools. This will perhaps have a greater effect than anything else on improving efficiency through saving time and reducing levels of frustration and irritation, and ensuring that management is properly informed about operational issues and constraints.

Patient information

The increasing interest of the general public in their own health will foster the development of general health educational resources. Primary and emergency care information and tools will be extended into the living room of every household. Information about health service providers and agencies, and about the nature, style, cost and quality of their work will be available on-line to assist with making personal care decisions.

Lifelong patient records

Patient held medical records (PHMR) devices will facilitate better lifelong patient records. They will store and/or index all significant health events for the holder. They will provide the private key which will enable authorised providers to identify an individual as well as to locate and access any relevant parts of his/her records stored both on the device as well as in remote locations (see wide area networks). Few people will wish to be without their own PHMR because of the improved speed, continuity and integrity of care that they promote.

Multimedia medical records

Most records will be stored in electronic form, although not all of the information will necessarily be classified and coded. Text based records will progressively give way to multimedia records, incorporating pictures, images and sketches, moving images, audio notes and memoranda, as well as text. All of these elements will be able to be recorded and replayed using point and click devices (such as mouse or trackball).

Display devices

Large and intrusive cathode ray screens will be replaced by flat colour displays (of any size) consuming much less power and generating virtually no electromagnetic field. Handheld "palmtop" computers will be radio-linked in to networks to provide mobile processing: flat "tablet" or pad computers with writing recognition capability will be widely used for data entry and retrieval. Much data will be recorded using check boxes, picking lists and agreed protocols. Voice recognition and electronic generation of clinical notes from dictation is still a way off: even when it arrives, it is likely to be cumbersome and unwieldy, and probably not the utopian dream that some are hoping for.

3

Clinical support

The mass of biomedical information from the world literature will be brought together into forms and tools that make it more readily accessible and usable. Endorsed and recommended approaches to the care of specific categories of patient ("best quality practices") will be available in computerised forms and will be continuously updated as new discoveries are made.

Movement of information

Wide area networking

National and international health communications networks are being developed. These will permit care providers to identify individuals and assemble their medical notes from wherever they are stored anywhere in the world. An authorised provider will be able to access records for his/her patients from the car, at the scene of an accident, in an aircraft, at home or anywhere via satellite or radio. Connection points will be wherever you want them: fixed in your home and office, or as mobile as a cell phone.

The same networks will enable you to order tests and receive results much faster, to find a bed for a patient, to make appointments for clinics, and to access an enormous range of important information.

Telemedicine

Distance from care facilities need no longer be an obstacle to the provision of best quality healthcare services. Remote monitoring of patients at home or anywhere else can be carried out over the telephone connections, so making frequent monitoring cost-effective and eliminating the inconvenience of unnecessary visits to the clinic. Remote consultations should become relatively commonplace, often with specialists who may be in their own homes. A difficult image or specimen may be reviewed and reported on in seconds by an expert, perhaps in another country. Waiting for an expert opinion will become unnecessary.

Interconnected systems

The technology to interconnect many different computer systems, for example within a hospital, is already available. This is often a rather ad hoc arrangement at present, but the next generation of systems will incorporate greatly improved standardised interfaces. For the first time purchasers will be able to mix and match the best available applications for their purposes, and to interface laboratory or intensive care monitoring equipment, for example, directly into their information systems backbone. Vendors will be distinguished on the basis of the functionality and services they provide rather than the hardware platform or technology they adopt.

Infrastructure developments

Most of the above developments presuppose that a range of essential infrastructure elements are implemented. Standards are needed for communications and messages, and for medical records structures and codes. Standards will also emerge for the style and operation of user interfaces, all but eliminating the time and effort required to learn how to use each new application. International identifiers for patients, providers, purchasers and care organisations will make it easy to communicate, exchange data, and reach agreements for the provision and payment for services. Most important of all, there will be a wide range of available resources for informatics education, orientation and skills development, often disseminated through distance learning techniques, creating a class of knowledgeable consumers of the new technologies.

Virtual environments

Our present view of the world is dominated by those with whom we interact and from whom we receive support, assistance and advice. Physical proximity has inevitably played a large part in this, since the speed and ease of interaction with people nearby is much greater and therefore the satisfaction is higher. Therefore our world has been dominated by those with whom we come into contact at work, at home, at play and through travel. But an increasing proportion has been contributed by telecommunication, through the telephone, journals and so on.

One of the big changes of the next decade or two will be the emergence of an entire range of virtual environments, from virtual conferences to virtual consultations and even virtual hospitals. The professional isolation that is experienced by so many professionals working away from the population centres will be largely a thing of the past, since they will be just as able to keep up-to-date, take part in interactive exchanges, have access to on-line knowledge bases and expertise as anyone anywhere in the world. Telecommuting will really take off, and broad band technology will make image transmission as ubiquitous as facsimile is today. Video mail (moving image and sound messages) will play an increasingly important role in routine work environments. The physical location of persons and resources will no longer be any sort of obstacle to quick, convenient, frequent and cheap access to them. Co-location of people and services (such as a hospital) will no longer be necessary.

The present state

Unfortunately, the state of information management in the health sector today is to be deplored. In 1990 the UK National Audit Office reported that the use of computers in the NHS had fallen far behind that in comparable businesses. By contrast, the business environment has been transformed by the implementation of computerised information systems over the past two decades. In the US, the proportion of that nation's total capital base represented by information systems rose from 7 per cent in 1980 to 14 per cent in 1991. Why has so little been achieved in the health sector whilst other sectors of the economy have forged ahead in harnessing the benefits of automation?

Before analysing some of the causes, we must first dismiss two of the issues that are often blamed but are definitively **not** the cause of the problem. These are availability of funds, and the capability of technology.

Funds

Investment in information systems by hospitals is remarkably low. Consider the following:

- The cost of a new hospital such as the Chelsea and Westminster Hospital is over £300 million (approx. US$ 475 million), but the purchases of healthcare computer systems and related services by NHS hospitals during the year 1992–93 came to only £220 million (approx. US$350 million) (source Silicon Bridge Research)
- At the UK Inland Revenue, expenditure on IT is now 20 per cent of their staff costs: the respective figure for the NHS is about 1 per cent
- Half of all UK GPs use a computer on their consulting room desk, while less than one in every hundred hospital doctors has access to a computer at the time he or she sees each patient

Technology

We have seen spectacular increases in the power and performance of computers. The desk-top personal computer today is as powerful as a mainframe of 15 years ago, and the hardware industry continues to provide machines that provide double the performance for about half the cost every 2 years.

Over the past decade

- Networking technology has advanced to provide robust and stable local and wide area environments
- Specifications for open (e.g. OSI) and proprietary linkages between systems permit most hardware platforms to be linked together at moderate cost
- Electronic data interchange protocols (such as EDIFACT) have been developed and are widely used in the commercial sector
- High level programming languages and environments have been developed which permit applications to be created and changed quickly and efficiently

It is difficult to identify any technical obstacles that significantly impede the development of appropriate healthcare systems and solutions. This statement should not be misinterpreted: it does not mean that all the pieces for building an effective health information system are readily available — they are not, and nor are the people who must be involved in the change necessarily culturally ready or sufficiently technically aware. However, the technology required for healthcare systems development is certainly available and has been in most instances for several years.

The obstacles

Several major issues have played a role in this remarkably slow development. Until they are addressed progress will remain slow. These include:

- Failure to place a market value on healthcare information; lack of a defined health information economy that acts to promote investment of private capital
- An inability by managers to perceive the benefits that could be derived from accurate, timely and comprehensive information
- Difficulty with addressing the cultural and attitude changes which information systems introduce into the workplace
- Ignorance of information technology amongst health personnel, both clinical and managerial; technophobia, and suspicion of automation
- Lack of the knowledge, understanding and skills needed to plan, procure and implement information systems successfully; lack of shared understanding between vendors and purchasers
- Lack of reference sites and demonstrators
- The size of the task required to put in place the informatics infrastructure, and absence of standards
- Lack of mutual understanding and alienation between clinicians, managers and information services personnel
- Difficulty in cost-justifying investment in technology, in part arising out of a belief that the costable benefits of computers are confined to clerical productivity
- Lack of effective national health informatics leadership and education over many years

Standards

Successful development of the health information environment requires minimised barriers to entry, both real and imagined, physical and conceptual. There is no benefit to the community in reinventing the wheel. It is counter-productive and costly. The only future for development of the health information environment, locally, nationally and globally, is through collaboration and adoption of common infrastructure standards.

Few users have any intrinsic interest in standards: they are not an issue that fire most people with excitement, but they are an absolutely fundamental element of the infrastructure, both as regards functionality and cost.

There are always several different ways of achieving the same end. For example, you could make a three-pin power plug in any number of configurations, and the international arena has a wide range of good examples. The problem arises when one person wants to plug their equipment into another type of socket, or when a vendor wants to manufacture equipment that can be sold to more than one purchaser. There is nothing wrong with an island as long as you are happy remaining on the island, cut off from everywhere else.

Flexibility and connectivity

But whilst island thinking still pervades much decision making, there is not the slightest doubt in the minds of those decision makers that the future lies in development of all sorts of interchanges and interactions, especially electronic. Whilst within your island environment you may choose to do things any way you wish, but when we come to establishing links between islands there are just two options:

1. Bespoke adaptors or "interfaces": one to match your plug with my socket, and a second to match my plug with your socket
2. Universal adaptors which designate an intermediary "standard", and then require end-users to build interfaces to and from that standard

What's the difference?

The bespoke option:

*   Requires 2 interfaces to link 2 environments/machines
*   Requires 6 interfaces to link 3 environments/machines
*   Requires 12 interfaces to link 4 environments/machines
*   Requires $n(n-1)$ interfaces to link n environments (e.g. 2450 for 50)

The bespoke option provides a formidable barrier to evolutionary development, because any change to one system (such as the use of an enhanced coding system) may require changes to all (n) systems connected to it. These changes would normally have to be done by the developers of these systems.

The standard option:

*   Requires 4 interfaces to link 2 environments/machines
*   Requires 6 interfaces to link 3 environments/machines
*   Requires 8 interfaces to link 4 environments/machines
*   Requires $2n$ interfaces to link n environments (e.g. 100 for 50)

The standard option facilitates evolution, because a change to one system should only require a single set of changes to maintain compliance with the standard. These changes would only affect the developers of the system being changed. Similarly a new system can be introduced at minimum cost, requiring only two interfaces—(to and from the standard).

Taking the first step into standards, may be more expensive but thereafter it is savings all the way down the line. That is the bottom line argument for standards, and it all depends upon whether you have the vision of the future, or not!

Other benefits from standardisation include:

- Ease of interchange of staff — standards allow staff to move easily from one work environment to another without the need to retrain
- Cost of purchases and support — any vendor can provide standard compliant equipment and any service person can maintain it; barriers to free competition are reduced
- Ability to mix and match — you can mix one standard component with any other to achieve the best match to your requirements; you are not restricted to the offerings of any one vendor
- Flexibility — you can pick the technology that fits best; there is no need to be locked in to "old" or obsolescent technology because of the non-standard nature of your installation.

There is also a potential downside to standards. Once a standard has been specified it becomes "the way", even if it emerges that it is not the best way. Standards may help unify the environment, but they can also pose an obstacle to future development. Standards also cost money to implement. Many enterprises have already invested once in developing their proprietary systems: they resent then being asked to buy a standard that basically achieves the same end, and so may charge more for standards-compliant equipment.

What is a standard?

A standard is a document providing rules, guidelines and specifications for devices, processes, activities or their results which are the subject of common and repeated use. Standards are established by consensus, approved by a recognised body aimed at the achievement of a maximum degree of order in a given context.

This definition is deliberately broad, but warrants rereading. Note that standards are intended to achieve order in things for common and repeated use. Another keyword is consensus, which is defined as general agreement, characterised by the absence of sustained opposition to substantial issues by any important part of the concerned interests, and by a process which involves seeking to take into account the views of all parties concerned and to reconcile any conflicting arguments. Note that consensus need not imply unanimity.

In healthcare computing the recognised body in Europe is CEN TC251. This technical committee was set up in 1990 with the scope and responsibility for the organisation, coordination and monitoring of the development of standards for healthcare informatics, as well as the promulgation of these standards. TC251 has established seven working groups:

1. Healthcare modeling and medical records
2. Semantics and knowledge representation
3. Communications and messages
4. Images and multimedia
5. Medical devices
6. Security, privacy, quality and safety
7. Intermittently-connected devices (such as smart-cards)

In each European country the national standards organisation has set up a local committee to feed into CEN TC251. In the UK, BSI has established Technical Committee IST/35 for the collection of views and the dissemination of information about standards in healthcare computing. In the United States, ANSI (American National Standards Institute) has set up the Health Informatics Standards Planning Panel (HISPP) to coordinate the work being done by various standards groups (including IEEE, HL7, ASTM, ACR/NEMA and X.12).

What sorts of standards are being developed?

Inter-operability — the ability of two different systems to work together, to interconnect and exchange information. There is a growing interest in networking, electronic messaging, file and document interchange; a range of key issues are emerging, such as the need for distributed processing within networks and for resource directories applicable to networked environments

Security and privacy — this is a high priority area for health information systems. It is apparent that existing approaches cannot provide the necessary balance between ease and flexibility of data access with the necessary levels of personal privacy protection

Applications portability — efforts are being channeled into the development of portable software environments (such as POSIX) which would permit applications developed in one environment to be ported onto other platforms which better meet users needs in terms of size, cost etc.

User interfaces — the variability of the human-computer interface across different software applications is a source of user confusion. Standardisation in this area could have a substantial impact on productivity, especially where, as in the health environment, users need to use a large number of different applications

Electronic Data Interchange — covers the messaging and communications environment required to support the growth in interworking between systems.

Electronic interchange of other file types — such as of audio files (heart sounds, breath sounds, voice mail etc.) and of image files (ECG, EEG, X-ray, cine-angiography etc.), to create full interchangeable multi-media environments

Health information classification and coding systems — the sheer number and complexity of classification and coding systems in common use in the health sector makes it especially difficult for computer systems to interwork, and for meaningful exchanges of data

Portable health records devices — the potential for smart cards and other portable devices to improve care through better data accessibility, whilst ensuring personal privacy makes such devices attractive, but a standard interface and data structure is needed to permit such devices to be used with any make or model of information system

Chapter 2   Historical milestones

History of healthcare Computing

The history of health sector computing has been chequered and inconsistent: there have been outstanding achievements, as well as abject failures. The latter have achieved the greater notoriety, and there is a long and sad catalogue of cases where large sums invested in hopeless developments have had to be written off. Even after 30 years of active development, there is not a single hospital anywhere in the world where computer systems provide anything that approaches the expectations of clinicians and managers. Simplistic explanations, such as lack of funding, will not do since healthcare services throughout the developed world continue to invest huge sums of money in new buildings and medical equipment.

In this chapter we have selected eight developments which we feel have been historically important. We do not suggest that these are the only important developments, simply that they seem to us to have influenced thinking and directions.

Four "early" developments

Medical applications have led to pioneering work in computer science, with many of the ideas developed initially for healthcare applications being subsequently adopted by the wider computing community. One example is the MUMPS language, which was originally developed at the Massachusetts General Hospital during the mid-1960s, and has since become widely used in healthcare and in commerce. Four other key landmarks specific to the early development of healthcare computing were the OXMIS, PROMIS, MYCIN and HELP which are outlined briefly below.

OXMIS

The Oxford Community Health Project (also called OXMIS), led by John Perry, pioneered the use of computers in general practice during the early 1970s. A mainframe computer held registration and encounter records for more than 100 GPs, generating epidemiological data (as well as providing direct benefits to the GPs). It was clear that the project required unambiguous coded data and its lasting claim to fame is the development of the OXMIS Codes.

The OXMIS Codes were the first comprehensive codes for primary care and preceded the development of the Read Codes (see below) by at least ten years. The OXMIS codes were based on ICD-8 and as late as 1993 were still being used by over 5000 GPs. The unfortunate illness and early death of John Perry meant that the OXMIS Codes were never developed further. Had this not happened there might have been no Read Codes, and OXMIS Version 2 would be the NHS standard for clinical codes.

PROMIS

Problem Oriented Medical Information System (PROMIS) was one of the first "paperless" clinical information systems used in a hospital. It was developed by Lawrence Weed, as a computer-based implementation of his concept of Problem Oriented Medical Records (POMR). The basic concept of the POMR is that clinical information should be recorded in relation to the problem to which it is relevant. Each patient should have a problem list, and each identified problem should have its own clinical findings, orders and decisions.

PROMIS also endeavoured to couple knowledge found in textbooks and libraries with the information known about the individual patient. Weed recognised that the quality of medical decision making was dependent upon the knowledge that the doctor had memorised and could retrieve from memory in the context of the specific patient.

PROMIS was designed to guide the doctor in reaching decisions through a sequence of screens designed for the systematic gathering of clinical information: each screen was called up as a consequence of the data entered in previous screens. In other words, the user is linked in to a structure of logical pathways embedded in the computer in the form of a medical knowledge base.

During the 1980s this has led on to the development of what Larry Weed has called "Problem-knowledge couplers". These couplers aim to guide the physician to collect the data that is required to reach a decision, and provide an analysis of the collected data for decision support. Couplers are now available for a range of presenting problems and situations.

MYCIN

MYCIN was an early attempt to develop an expert system for the selection of an appropriate antibiotic in patients with meningitis and blood infections. The system was developed by Ed Shortliffe, at the

University of Stanford in America. The system comprises a large number of production rules, each of which constitutes a statement of the "if (antecedents) then (consequents)" type. Evaluation of the system demonstrated significant support for it: they confirmed its ability to perform at a level similar to that of an infectious diseases expert and at least as well as staff of the medical faculty.

Although it was not routinely used in the clinical setting, various expert systems that followed it were able to gain sufficient user acceptance to be useful clinically. However, although more than 1000 medical expert systems have been developed to date, few have ever gained widespread acceptance despite demonstrations of their capacity to perform at least as well as doctors.

HELP

The HELP system pioneered many of the issues involved in bringing decision support systems into the clinical workplace. It grew out of early work by Homer Warner at the University of Utah on the use of computers to enhance clinical decision-making. By the late 1970s the system was installed throughout all departments of the hospital, and made use of a common database for all clinical services.

The HELP system was an early hospital information system, but the unique feature of this system has been the implementation of logic in a modular fashion. Simple medical decision logic modules (MDLMs) are of the "if . . . then . . ." type, and these may be linked together into complex trees. A module may be invoked by, for example, the ordering of an investigation, the decision to prescribe a drug, or by another logic module that calls upon it. The output from the MDLMs can go to providing interpretations of data, indicating logical follow-on from an investigation, or to generating reports and alarms where attention may be required.

The value of the system for clinicians was evaluated and indicated that they were supportive because, amongst other reasons:

- The data was better organised than in written notes
- Useful interpretative data was provided by the logic modules
- Attention was focused on important issues
- Computer-performed calculations were an asset
- Speed of communications between departments was enhanced
- Redundant data collection was eliminated
- Computer-generated medication schedules for each patient and shift helped nurses and minimised errors

Recent work has led to the development of a standardised way of representing the information to be included in MDLMs (the "Arden" syntax), and the beginnings of the development of a library of MDLMs for use by systems developers.

More recent Computing landmarks

More recent clinical computing developments have concentrated on creating the necessary infrastructure for communication and exchange of patient care information. Four key landmark developments have been selected, each of which is prototypic. These are the Read Clinical Classification system, the Exeter Care Card project, the New Zealand National Health Information System, and the QMR (Quick Medical Reference) medical knowledge base.

Read codes

A large number of classification and coding systems have been developed and are in current usage for different purposes. There are classifications of diseases (e.g. ICD), of primary care activities, of medication, of occupation, of procedures (e.g. OPCS, CPT), of pathology (e.g. SNOP) and much more. The special contribution of the Read Codes has been to bring these together into a single system that provides for all the needs of clinicians, whether in primary, secondary or tertiary care.

The Read Codes were originally conceived by James Read, then a general practitioner in Loughborough, as a means of keeping track of the preventive care of his patients. This required only a very small number of codes. However, through its use the benefits of a more comprehensive system for computerised records became clear, and by the late 1980s it had expanded to a system that provided for the majority of the needs of general practice.

Recognising that the Read Codes were unlikely to replace all other healthcare coding systems, each of which retains its own niche in the health sector to which it is particularly well suited, the Read Codes have been developed with a set of utilities for code conversions. This means that data recorded in Read Codes can be translated and reported in most of the other major classification systems, so enabling them to coexist productively side-by-side. The Read system is described in greater detail in chapter 9.

Care card

The NHS Care Card project (launched in 1989) demonstrated the practicality of using portable electronic devices (in this instance the device was a smart card) to transport personal health records. Initially some 8,000 patients living in the Exmouth area (south-west England) were supplied with cards: the number was subsequently doubled. Local general practitioners, dentists, pharmacists and the hospital casualty department were supplied with equipment to read and write to the cards. Records of care encounters and decisions, including prescriptions, were written to the card so that other providers of care were made more aware of the patients' various healthcare encounters.

This was one of the first successful attempts to overcome the

15

growing problem of record fragmentation. In the NHS, record fragmentation is perhaps slightly less than in other systems because each patient is assigned to a primary care provider (GP). Even so there are significant problems in ensuring that information is shared efficiently between the growing number of professionals who constitute the team caring for a patient, and especially those with chronic and complex problems.

In other countries, where each individual has the right to select their care provider for each and every encounter, the complex network of care interactions results in a proliferation of partial records for each individual and a much greater fragmentation of the medical record for each person. Inevitably this affects the integrity and continuity of care provided to the individual.

New Zealand national health information system

The New Zealand Health Information Service has implemented the first stage of a national health information network for health information interchange between care sector personnel. The special features of this system, which went live in mid-1993, are:

- A national unique personal identifier for healthcare purposes, served from a central file server, with comprehensive protection for personal information privacy
- A national electronic health event/encounter report collection system
- A network based on open system (OSI) compliance
- A point of connection for all care personnel, with the minimum of constraints on equipment requirements
- A national health communications network based on Value Added Network (VAN) service providers
- Selected messages specified and based on HL7 (interactive) and EDIFACT (batch) communications protocols

The first phase of this development used public funds to create an infrastructure and incentives to make use of the system. This is now attracting private capital to provide further functionality and applications (e.g. order communications, booking of admissions and appointments etc.) for primary and secondary care providers.

QMR medical knowledge base

The QMR knowledge base constitutes the first comprehensive knowledge base developed specifically for health professionals. The QMR system was developed at the University of Pittsburgh by profiling specified internal medicine conditions in terms of the patterns of clinical findings that may be present. The sources of the data are cited, and are drawn largely from the published literature.

Two indices assist the user. Each finding is assigned a value for the "evoking strength", that is the degree to which that finding would lead one to think in terms of each possible condition. A second value, called the "frequency", indicates how often that finding would be present in a patient known to be suffering from a nominated condition.

At one level this is a dynamic electronic textbook of medicine, providing a useful educational resource. At another level the system can be used to assist in diagnosis, and especially in the diagnosis of patients where there may be two or more coincident problems. It can critique a proposed diagnosis and can suggest ways to distinguish between a list of differential diagnoses.

IM&T strategy for the NHS

The NHS Information Management and Technology (IM&T) Strategy was launched in December 1992. It is intended to provide a foundation for electronic exchange of information throughout the NHS. The Strategy covers all aspects of the NHS including acute and non-acute hospital care, community care, primary care, commissioners and support services.

The IM&T Strategy is based on the business goal of the NHS Executive to create a better health service for the nation in three ways:

1. Ensuring services are of highest quality and responsive to needs and wishes of patients. The intention is to provide seamless personal care so that relevant medical history and test results are available whenever and wherever they are needed

2. Ensuring that health services are effectively targeted so as to improve the health of local populations

3. Improving efficiency of services so that as great a volume of well targeted and effective services as possible is provided from available resources. To achieve efficient use of resources, investments must be appraised and benefits realised.

The vision

The IM&T Strategy's vision is to support better care and communication. The vision is of an NHS where, subject to security and confidentiality safeguards, information is shared by all those who can benefit from it — for example, hospitals, GP practices, community care, dentists, pharmacists, district health authorities (DHAs) and Family Health Service Authorities (FHSAs) — and is available when and where it is needed. Patients should benefit through increased efficiency, accuracy and timeliness of information. Staff should use the information from these systems for patient care, but also for quality audit and continuous quality improvement of the service(s) they provide.

Implementation

The Strategy sets out a framework for implementation of computer systems throughout the NHS between now and the year 2000, by when all large hospitals should have fully *integrated*[1] electronic information systems. It is designed to be implemented at three levels: central, regional and local.

Centrally, the Information Management Group (IMG) of the NHS Executive (NHS ME) sets policy and standards and disseminates good practice. Each NHS Region co-ordinates implementation of the IM&T infrastructure within its region and approves capital investments for information systems costing in excess of £1 million. At the local level, teams of managers, clinicians and IM&T staff at each NHS Trust are required to develop a local strategy and action plans that comply with national standards. Purchasing and implementation of computer systems is a local decision and each hospital is expected to choose whatever systems it needs according to its own priorities and needs.

Key principles

The key principles behind the Strategy are:

1. Information systems are to be person-based, with a separate healthcare record for each patient, referenced by that person's NHS number
2. Computer systems should interwork, so that, wherever practical, data is entered on a computer once only. Subsequently, that information may be made available as required by other systems
3. Information should be derived from operational systems used by doctors and other healthcare professionals in their day-to-day work; there should be little need for separate systems to capture management information, although they will be required to process and report it.
4. Care must be taken to ensure that information held on computers is only available to those with a need to know and who are authorised to know it.

---

[1] The word *integrated* should be used with caution. In the IM&T Strategy it really means *interfaced*, so that various systems in the hospital can exchange information with no need for duplicate data entry.

5. Standards for healthcare data interchange, coding and NHS-wide networking are needed to allow computer-to-computer communication so that information can be shared between healthcare professionals in hospitals, GP practices and commissioning agencies.

This Strategy represents a significant move towards encouraging the implementation of operational systems, and away from the IT policy prevalent during the late 1970s and 1980s, which was oriented towards collecting management and administrative data.

Summary

These developments have put in place some of the building blocks on which future healthcare computing systems will be based:

- The need for unique identifiers has been recognised.
- The development of a user-friendly classification and coding system for all of healthcare has been initiated.
- The importance of linking clinical findings with knowledge and logical structures has been explored.
- The importance of systems that can support and critique decisions has been identified.
- Techniques for moving patient information both using networks and cards have been developed.

Much remains to be done, but these examples illustrate some of the key issues that must be incorporated in future systems developments.

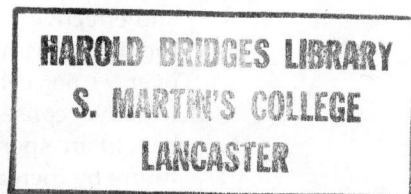

Chapter 3 Information, quality and decisions

Medicine is able to do more and more to care for individuals, but at a cost. That cost is steadily escalating, and the rate of increase shows no signs of slowing. As a result there are not sufficient resources available to go round: people must wait, or even go without. The slogan "health for all" seems no nearer to being achieved. We have to find ways of doing more for less, of improving the cost-effectiveness of the care system as a whole.

Decisions about care are made in the belief that those services selected have the best chance of improving the status of an individual or community, but in many cases there is little objective evidence to support current patterns of resource consumption.

The big picture

The healthcare system sets out to achieve its goals through two concurrent strategies. The first strategy is *preventive*: it sets out to reduce exposure to health risks. This is achieved through public health measures, paying attention to environmental pollution and to safety at home, at work and elsewhere. Susceptibility to many health risks is partly genetic, but can be modified by healthy lifestyles, immunisation programmes and so on, and hence there is a major role for health education and promotion activities within the preventive strategy.

The second strategy is *curative*: this sets out to minimise the impact, severity and duration of illnesses through early detection and effective treatment of identifiable problems. At the present time the budget is heavily biased towards curative care, which consumes over 99 per cent of the overall budget. This is probably one of the negative consequences of health politics: there is greater political benefit in spending more on acute care than in investing for the future by increasing the expenditure on preventive care. The benefits from preventive care programmes may often not be evident for 20–50 years after the interventions.

Healthcare goals and relationships

The goal of the healthcare system is to provide for the healthcare needs of the patients. The twin aims are often stated as the reduction of avoidable morbidity (illness) and of premature mortality (death). The vital issue that sometimes seems to get lost in the process of delivering care services is that the *patient* is the focus of the care effort. The patient is the consumer of the services, and therefore the goal must be to ensure that the needs, wishes and best interests of the patient are catered for.

However, the patient is not a customer in quite the way that the buyer of an electrical appliance is. The patient often does not know what he or she needs in the way of services, and often is only marginally involved in selecting the provider of services, especially when it comes to hospital care. The principal business relationship for the suppliers of hospital services is with the general practitioners who are the source of their patient referrals and are often referred to as the gatekeepers for access to the secondary care system.

Organisational domains

The organisation of healthcare delivery is split into primary, secondary and tertiary domains. Primary care refers to those who are the first point of contact with the patient. The bulk of primary care is at present delivered by general or family practitioners. Various other health professionals may have primary level contacts with patients, for example community care staff (nurses, midwives etc.), pharmacists and others. The primary care provider is a specialist in the wide range of human ailments: for those problems which need further analysis and treatment, the primary care provider acts as the gatekeeper to the next tier of the system (secondary care), and refers the patient on to the appropriate service(s) for further management.

Secondary care is normally accessed as a consequence of a referral from a primary care provider. The secondary care environment comprises the hospitals as well as the various specialist referral services which may be located outside hospitals (e.g. specialist physicians and surgeons in their rooms). Secondary care is widely referred to as if it comprised only inpatient (residential) acute care. However, many hospitals provide services which do not require the admission of the patient. For example, there are outpatient clinics, accident and emergency services, day case services and various analytical, diagnostic and laboratory services. These may be variously classified in the primary/secondary division depending more on politics and organisational structures than on semantic integrity. For outpatient and day case care a referral is normally required from primary care. However, accident and emergency is based on self-referral: similarly, many ambulatory care services may have significant numbers of walk-in or unplanned patients, some of whom may have been patients of the service at some previous time.

Tertiary care is practically indistinguishable from secondary care in that it uses the same plant, personnel and resources. Tertiary care is accessed by a referral from secondary care, and it may often involve a greater degree of complexity or sophistication. However, secondary and tertiary care patients share all the same facilities.

All providers, whatever the domain they come from, generate costs by requesting further services for their patients. These may be requests for tests and investigations, orders for medications or appliances, referrals for further consultations or procedures, and so on. The system can only function effectively and efficiently if this process is organised and well managed. These decisions generate further costs for the patient (or whoever is paying for the services), as well as exposing the patient to risks (every service, however trivial, carries some degree of risk). Clearly only those services where the potential benefit outweighs the potential risks should be selected, and the only person in a position to make that decision is the care provider, who is responsible for that patient.

The organisational arrangement of the care system is a major determinant of the pattern and quality of care and services delivered to patients. The present arrangement is widely perceived as being a problem in itself, and the process of business re-engineering seeks to replace this structure with something better serving the goals of the service, and the needs of the patients.

Care integrity

A gulf has grown up between the organisational domains of the healthcare system, especially between primary and secondary care. The patients are common to both, but in other respects the domains share very little in common. Secondary and tertiary care together have progressively consumed a growing proportion of the health budget, and at the same time have come to have greater influence over health politics than the primary care sector. This despite the fact that a very large proportion of the population have primary care encounters in any one year, but only a very small proportion progress on to secondary care events. The gatekeeping role of the GP is difficult to execute if the data is not available to them.

This has led to the development of *Managed Care* plans. In broad terms, managed care is a plan whereby the general practitioner manages and tracks the patient through all his/her encounters with primary, secondary and tertiary care services, retaining overall responsibility for the provision of services. This is in contrast to the prevalent alternative where responsibility for a patient is passed from one provider to another: in this latter arrangement, patients can "fall through the cracks" between services and suffer as a consequence.

However, this gulf between primary and secondary care has become a major obstacle to communication and to total quality management (see below), making it difficult to implement managed care plans. There is distrust between the staff of the two domains, as well as a degree of physical separation. General practitioners resent the attitude of superiority of many secondary care providers, which seems to be evidenced by inadequate and untimely communications as well as lack of consideration for each other. Patients come from and return to the communty where they are the on-going responsibility of primary and community care services: their stay in hospital is normally just a short and small part of their overall illness.

The need to place the needs of the patient first is paramount. The need for sharing the care of the patient between providers from primary and secondary care is self-evident. Much of the difficulty in achieving this results from lack of understanding and poor communication.

Clinical and administrative information

Everyone wants the health service to provide economical and effective patient care by providing quality services which are timely and efficient. In considering these issues, we treat the health service as having two separate functions: service management and clinical care.

Service management covers all those parts of the health service responsible for providing routine services such as laboratory tests, procedures, meals and so on. These services need to be produced and delivered to an appropriate quality at minimum cost, that is to say as efficiently as possible.

The second function, **clinical care**, is dominated by the process of gathering information and using it to make clinical decisions for each individual patient. These decisions involve the consumption of resources (e.g. tests, procedures, medications, appliances, periods of hospitalisation etc.) required for diagnosis and management.

If you doubt the depth of the division between service management and clinical practice, consider the day-to-day operation of a private hospital, where the split is most obvious. The management of the hospital is responsible for providing the hotel, nursing and other services, while the consultant is the customer for these services, acting as an agent for the patient.

Over the years managers have made repeated but ultimately misguided attempts to equate their own information needs with those of doctors. Hospital activity analysis in the mid 1970s, "Korner" data sets in the early 1980s, resource management in the late 1980s and now contract management systems have each in turn been trumpeted as systems which would help doctors and improve patient care. That these ideas should have been put forward on the basis of honest beliefs reveals an almost incredible gulf in understanding of what doctors do, and their information needs.

For patients with similar diseases, age and sex, more than 80 per cent of variance in the cost of care can be explained by differences in clinical practice, that is, doctors' patterns of treatment and investigation. Less than 20 per cent of variance in costs is attributable to the hospital itself, the efficiency with which service departments carry out specified services. These figures come from US research where costs of healthcare have been analysed using analysis of variance techniques. Work in the NHS by the Audit Commission on pathology services, day surgery and use of medical beds has demonstrated enormous variations in practices and patterns of care which point to a comparable situation in the UK.

Differing clinical practices reflect the differing clinical decision making processes and preferences of individual doctors. These, in turn, are dependent on their clinical knowledge bases, experiences, attitudes, expertise and training. Clinical decisions are made on the basis of confidence, which in turn is based on information: information in the head of the decision-maker, information on paper in the patient notes and records, and information that is made available in other forms such as on computer screens.

Quality management

The principles of Total Quality Management (TQM) are:

- Attention to the process of healthcare delivery
- Commitment to the consumer of care services
- Involvement of the staff in management
- Identification of best practice

The keys to successful implementation of TQM include:

- Promotion of a customer focus — perceiving the patient's, GP's or purchaser's view of the services on offer
- Visible involvement and backing for TQM from the chief executive and senior management
- Linking the TQM focus to clear strategic goals, such as improving customer satisfaction, reducing delays, cutting costs, improving service quality
- Linking TQM to financial payback and ensuring that improved quality performance delivers measurable benefits

Patients may continue to put up with poor service, bad behaviour, inconvenience and distress if they perceive that this is ultimately to the betterment of their health, but none would choose this preferentially. For too long health services have managed to avoid being held accountable to their consumers.

The traditional fabric of healthcare is changing fast. Hospitals are being downsized as a result of moving care services into the community, so reducing lengths of inpatient care and promoting development of care protocols that are patient focused and more clinically effective. Closer co-operation and improved communications are being established between primary and secondary care. Standards of service, patient comfort and convenience are now priority issues.

Information and decisions

At every level in the care system decisions have to be taken. At the highest levels, decisions are made about health policy and strategies, and about funding of programmes and building of facilities. At the level of the purchasers of care services, decisions have to be made about prices, contracts and performance of provider units. At the level of a service unit (primary, secondary or tertiary), decisions about business and clinical directions, and about efficiency and effectiveness of services must be made. At the level of the individual patient and provider, decisions about the services required for cost-effective care must be made. Every decision requires accurate, adequate and timely information.

Sources of health information

Traditional healthcare information systems address only a small part of this whole. Information is gathered mainly from the hospital sector, focusing on selected quantitative issues such as numbers of admissions, bed days, staff, costs and so on. Little is known about the health status and needs of the vast majority of the community who are not inpatients. Nor is much known about the appropriateness, quality, effectiveness or outcome of any of the care services provided.

Healthcare purchasers

Purchasers are responsible for the health of any community or region, and need to ensure that the services they purchase are:

- Appropriate to the community needs and act to improve community health status
- Of appropriate quality and performed with due care and skill
- Provided in a timely manner that is satisfactory to both patient and purchaser
- Provided in conformity with relevant legislation
- Carried out by appropriately skilled, experienced, qualified and registered persons
- Effective for the purposes, and achieving the desired outcome
- Offered at an attractive (contracted) price
- Accounted for through the provision of appropriate information

Health status monitoring

The health status of the community is affected by strategies to reduce the risks of premature death and avoidable illness (proactive and preventive care), as well as services provided to treat those who become ill (reactive and curative care). Individual health status is

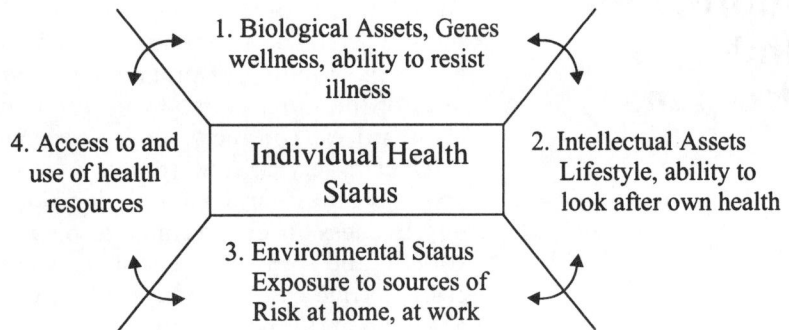

```
                    1. Biological Assets, Genes
                       wellness, ability to resist
                              illness

4. Access to and     ┌─────────────────────┐      2. Intellectual Assets
   use of health     │   Individual Health │         Lifestyle, ability to
   resources         │        Status       │         look after own health
                     └─────────────────────┘
                    3. Environmental Status
                       Exposure to sources of
                       Risk at home, at work
```

Figure 3.1

complex, but comprises principally four interlinked factors. They are:

1. **Biological status** — wellness and ability to resist illness (inherited factors, immune status etc.)
2. **Knowledge and intellectual status** — ability to look after own health and well-being, lifestyle
3. **Environmental exposure** — risks, pollution and hazards at home, work etc.
4. **Consumption of health resources** — access and intelligent usage, screening etc.

Note that a change in any one of these factors very often leads to a concomitant change in one or more of the others: for example those with greater intellectual assets are often able to make better use of care services, and appropriate use of care services (e.g. immunisation) can improve the biological assets of the individual.

Healthcare service units

Managers of service provider units, such as hospitals, clinics and community services, have their own information needs, and in addition have to respond to the needs of their funders (purchasers).

Their own needs reflect the need to attract contracts and consumers for their services, and to satisfy purchasers with the quality and value for money of the services they provide. Winning and keeping business depends upon both clinical and administrative performance.

Service managers need information on:

- Business performance indicators (e.g. patient throughput, bed occupancy, waiting and delays, workloads) used to evaluate the efficiency of service provision and resource utilisation
- Clinical performance indicators to monitor effectiveness of service provision

- Costs of providing services, and profitability (e.g. supply contracts, average lengths of stay etc.)

Provider units need to establish their reputation based on reliable facts and figures. Purchasers will place business with units which offer value for money, and can substantiate superior performance claims. Performance data may soon have to be audited as a condition of contracting for healthcare services.

Provider units must obtain information systems that can support their clinical and business requirements. The consequences of not having this information available are bleak, and include loss of contracts, down-sizing and eventual closure.

Clinical decisions

Clinical decisions are made in relation to diagnosis, services and referrals, and treatment of the individual. The process of medical decision making has been extensively researched, but is still not fully elucidated. However, in broad terms the process appears to be as follows.

A patient brings their problem(s) to the provider. The provider rapidly develops a number of hypotheses as to the possible causes (an hypothesis list), and gradually refines these by asking questions and performing examinations. What is actually happening is that the perceived probability of the leading hypotheses as to the cause of this problem are being continuously reviewed in the light of the available data.

The provider then reaches a point where no further purpose is served by this encounter. Various possibilities as to the cause remain viable, and form a differential diagnosis list. Services are requested and/or referrals organised in order to reach a definitive diagnosis: alternatively if none of the possible causes seems to warrant further investigation, the patient may be managed symptomatically (e.g. a sore throat and runny nose being managed with aspirin without ever definitively identifying the diagnosis or causative agent).

Definitive diagnoses are reached by a mixture of strategies. However, the process is based on probabilities. No diagnosis ever reaches the level of absolute certainty — there is always room for doubt in medical matters. The doctor has a general perception (accurate or otherwise) of the *prior probability* that a specific diagnosis is the cause of the problem. After new items of information are gathered the probabilities are refined. Each data item gathered should contribute towards making one or other diagnosis more or less probable, or else it is a waste.

At some point the perceived probability is high enough for a decision on treatment to be taken. The success (or not) of this treatment may lead to a further cycle of data gathering and review of the diagnostic decision.

The process of probability manipulation is not a strong feature of

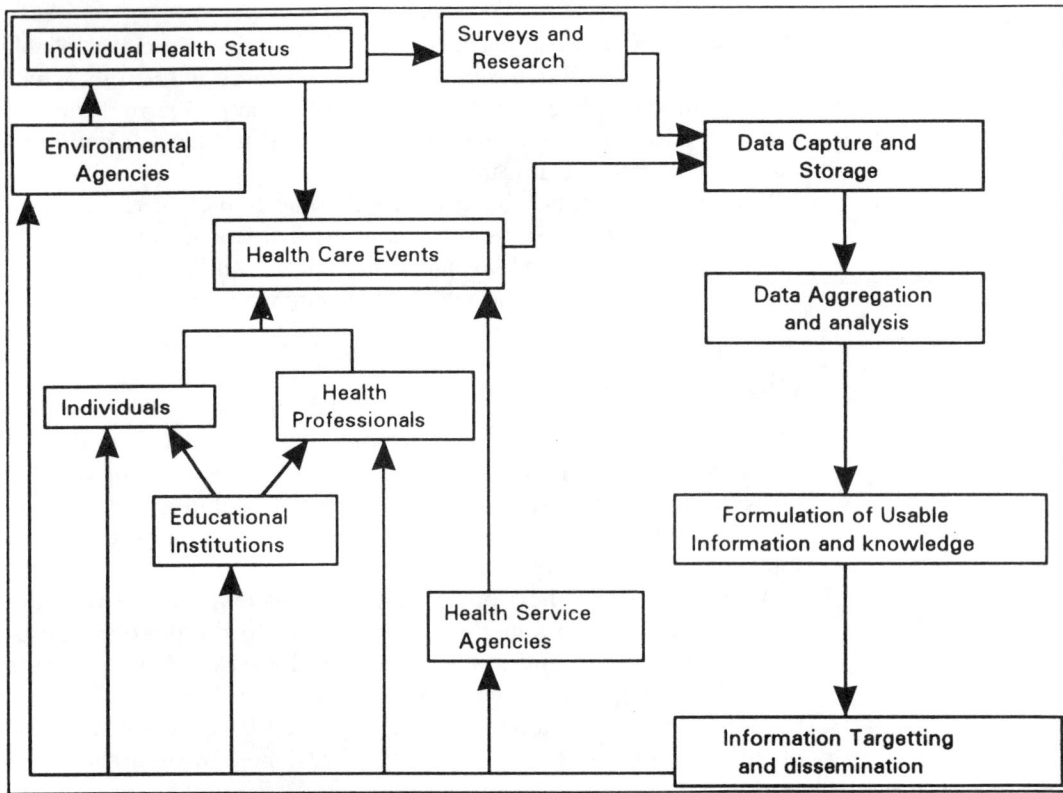

Figure 3.2 The "big picture" view of health information flow and management

human reasoning. However, given an appropriate knowledge base, computers can accurately calculate probabilities using Bayes Theorem. This is at the heart of many decision support and expert systems for use in medicine.

Linking through information systems

Purchasers and providers need to understand each other's aims and information requirements. Each tends to use information in two different ways.

The first is for *monitoring* of activity, for example, gathering data for administration, contract management and monitoring of business efficiency. The second is broader and involves, aiming to achieve *changes* by "closing the feedback loop". The future is based on change, on making better use of the existing health budget. Examples include changes in the organisation and delivery of services, in the behaviour of professionals and patients, and in the environmental factors which affect health status.

Sharing of information will help the various players to develop mutual understanding and to behave as partners. We need:

- Best quality practice protocols, agreed by purchasers and providers as the most cost-effective approach to providing preventive and curative care to certain categories of patient
- Patient-focused care protocols where the needs of the patient are the focal point of the services provided, and care is shared and co-ordinated between primary and secondary care
- New styles and patterns of health care practice and services delivery

The information economy

Information is power. Information is valuable and is an asset that must be worked hard. Provision of information has a cost, especially if it is comprehensive, accurate and timely, and provided in a specified form, such as a coded electronic message.

The health sector should explicitly recognise the value and the cost of information. We should separate the health budget into two parts: one is the market for services, where payments are made for the delivery of care services; the other is the market for information, where payment is made for the provision of information about health services, events and activities.

Justification of investment in information systems often comes down to explicit recognition of this fundamental issue. It is unrealistic to base investment appraisal for information systems mainly on potential for productivity improvements. Information costs money and has a value. Once that is accepted, investment appraisal is an exercise in market economics. If the information is wanted, for whatever reason, it must have a market price, and that determines how much one can afford to invest in systems to provide it. Market forces will then drive development: where there is a demand, fuelled by funds, there will soon be suppliers, and this applies to information as to any other commodity.

The advantages of a formalised health information economy are numerous. It indicates the importance of information, allowing developers and vendors to have confidence in the future of health information systems and therefore to justify serious investment. It allows for providers of information to be rewarded, so long as their information is accurate, adequate, timely and supplied in a form that is consistent with that required.

Imagine if the health information economy were defined as 10 per cent of the health economy. Purchasing authorities would allocate 90 per cent of the fee for each service to the provision of the service itself, and the remaining 10 per cent to the provision of information about the service. It would not be long before provider units were well equipped with information systems to maximise their income. There is no surer way to promote development of appropriate information systems than to specify precisely what information is required and how much it is worth when provided as specified.

The information cycle

The source of most data in the healthcare system is the notes and records that are made as a result of encounters between patients and health professionals. This encounter data should move through a variety of pathways to be assembled into information for different clinical and administrative purposes. Information so created should contribute to clinical and management decisions and in the longer term to the development of new knowledge. In other words there is, or should be, a cyclical movement of information whereby the raw data generated in care encounters is assembled into information which eventually finds its way back, directly or indirectly, to the participants in the care encounter.

This accumulated knowledge should improve the quality and outcomes of healthcare encounters by for example:

- Building up the clinical knowledge and understanding of the health professionals
- Identifying those management options that are more cost-effective
- Disseminating knowledge about availability, quality and cost of referral services
- Improving the ways in which care services are organised and presented to users
- Empowering users to interact productively with the care system
- Enabling patients to make informed decisions about alternative management options
- Enabling the community to identify and manage the risks to their own health

It is in this area that health information management systems at present have the least impact and the most potential. Some of the ways whereby this may come about are as outlined below.

Information when and where it is needed

Clinicians are concerned with the effective care of individual patients. Clinical practice generates vast amounts of data about individual patients. The cornerstone of the healthcare process is the consultation between a doctor and a patient. By the end of the consultation, either the doctor does or does not feel confident that he/she understands what is happening to the patient, based entirely on information available at the time. If the doctor is not confident about making a diagnosis he/she may order more tests to reduce uncertainty, or refer the patient to a colleague. Inevitably this creates further delays in treatment and extra costs of investigations and visits.

A national healthcare network could bring together the fragmented mini-records of a patient's record. This will lead to more accurate and comprehensive information, better and faster decisions, less duplication (e.g. of tests) and less risk of problems (e.g. interactions between medications given by different doctors at the same time). Recent test results will be available on-line by computer to the doctor as soon as the laboratory has completed the tests, rather than waiting for the mail.

Better organisation

Appointments and waiting lists can be computerised. Health professionals should see patients on time by appointment. Hospitals should be able to tell patients when they will be admitted. If a patient is referred on from one clinic to another, he or she should be able to choose when and where to go, and to make convenient arrangements there and then. Each doctor should know who each patient is and why they are there before they arrive — there should be no need to provide the same information time and time again.

Similarly laboratories should know what samples need to be collected, when and where, and which patients will be attending in person, when and for what, so that tests can be batched and run in the most efficient groups and times.

Greater convenience

The pressure of finances means that, especially in the less densely populated areas, there could be a tendency to reduce local services and move people to other locations for specialist work. However, the electronic network can bring full specialty services to every clinic, wherever located, using "Telemedicine" techniques. This permits links to be made when needed with specialists based elsewhere, not necessarily even in the same country, for long range consultations, diagnoses, opinions or for interpretation of test results or images. Rural communities will benefit greatly from the convenience of not having to make the journey to a far away specialist clinic. The political goal of equity of access to care and resources can be achieved in this way.

Some patients may not need to attend for an encounter in person, but could send information to the clinic over the telephone line. Telemonitoring of patients could eliminate large numbers of unproductive routine follow-up visits, and would allow even more frequent monitoring of identified high risk patients but without their needing to attend the hospital unless there is clear evidence of a problem.

Increased speed and efficiency

Increased speed of information movement will be of benefit not only in the clinical encounter, but also in administration. The financial processes will be greatly simplified through electronic handling. This should waste less time and ensure faster settlements. Greater overall efficiency of this process will result, so ensuring that less money is spent on financial administration and more is available for providing care services to individuals.

Informing doctors

Doctors find it difficult to keep up-to-date with information on recent developments in care procedures and techniques, especially when located some distance from the main population centres. The same network may be used to bring information to the professionals, to provide refresher courses and up-date materials as and when they find convenient, to be used and reused as often as required. The doctor may also find it difficult to know which of the local facilities provides required referral services, and how long the wait is, or where an acute care bed can be found at this very moment. All this information will be available on-line, and kept up-to-date all the time. Not only will doctors have clinical information at hand, but also the administrative details required to achieve a speedy resolution to each patient's problems. Some of these services may be a little time in development, but they are not too far away.

Informing managers

Most healthcare information relates to transactions (e.g. an admission, a service, an immunisation, a test result etc.). Individual transaction records may be important in TQM, but summaries and overviews are of the greatest significance to managers. The processes involved in gathering information should be directly aligned with those used for reporting/summarising the transactions. Managers will focus on the "outliers" which are identified as exceptions from normal ranges. A system which brings together information in this way, and displays it in graphical format for executives is called an Executive Information System (EIS). An EIS enables a manager quickly to identify trends and find exceptions, and then to "drill down" to the raw data to discover why they were exceptional.

These exceptions can often be grouped on the basis of membership of a specific community or population which is exposed to specific risks. Geographic Information Systems (GISs) enable data to be displayed in this way. Health and illness have geographic linkages, and it can be useful to display information about health events on the basis of domicile or workplace.

Informing patients

More and more people are taking an active interest in their own health and in managing it better. To do that they need access to the best advice on prevention as well as explanatory material about any illnesses that they or their relatives may suffer from and what options are available for their management. It is becoming increasingly important that individuals in the community feel empowered through information in order to make decisions about their own healthcare.

Better integrity of care

It will not be long before it is practical for individuals to carry their own health information with them. In practice, rather than carry the full details, the individual might carry an abstract containing the information most likely to be important (e.g. emergency care, medical warnings, current medications etc.), as well as a listing of where the other pieces of the medical record can be found. This would constitute a "key" which permits finding and retrieval of any computerised records belonging to you. For some people who travel extensively locally or overseas, or who are chronically ill and require the services of a large team of specialist providers, this might be a life-saver, or the key that frees them to travel when before they were afraid to go far from their local hospital.

Overall

Together these add up to a lot of good reasons for needing better healthcare information systems. The healthcare systems of the future will be based on wide area networks, and to add more value to the data that is gathered than happens at present. The need for information and knowledge to be presented in an appropriate form to the participants in the healthcare encounter is critical to improving the process and outcomes of healthcare.

Chapter 4   Computing basics

Information revolutions

Healthcare services are only now beginning to come to terms with the third great information revolution, based on the use of computers and electronic communications for the management of information.

The first information revolution came with the invention of writing several thousand years ago in the Middle East, which enabled permanent records to be kept for the first time. Before writing, information could only be held in human memory and much knowledge was inevitably lost whenever a person died. Modern healthcare, involving teams of specialist doctors and nurses, would be impossible without written records.

The second information revolution began with the invention of printing by Gutenberg in the 15th century. This provided, for the first time, the ability to replicate information without laborious transcription. The subsequent development of the printing and publishing industries has led to widespread availability of books and journals, transforming the dissemination of medical knowledge and medical education.

The essential nature of the information remained unchanged during this process. The information was static: its form and arrangement were determined at the time of its creation, and the tools for its navigation (e.g. contents list, index) were similarly predetermined, if present at all. The consequence is that it can be very hard to find just what you want in a bulky record, especially one that has no contents or index and is hand-written, as in the case of the traditional medical record.

The third revolution started some forty years ago with the development of electronic computers. The fundamental difference permitted by this change is that the information becomes dynamic, able to be organised and formatted according the wishes of its users. The use of electronic technology allows information to be disseminated faster and more widely, and eliminates the need for all the traditional impedimenta of the publishing world (typesetting, printing presses, binding etc.). The user can search and rearrange the information to suit their own needs and interests, and make as many copies as are required. The information can be available simultaneously in many locations, and can be moved rapidly between locations, and across borders without any effective barriers.

This revolution continues to gather pace as the costs of computers continue to fall and their power increases. Every ten years the power of computers (considered in terms of speed and storage capacity) increases by about a thousand fold. This extraordinary rate of development has continued now for forty years and shows no sign of slowing.

Representation of information

Over the centuries, the representation of information has become increasingly specific. The earliest way of representing information was by drawing a picture. The earliest writing was based on pictograms, which remains the basis of Chinese characters today. The cruciform characters of Mesopotamia were designed for the limitations of making indentations in clay tablets, and these ultimately led to the modern phonetically-based Greek and Latin alphabets. In English, all written information is represented by just 26 letters and 10 numerals. Whilst there are several other alphabets with differing numbers of characters, the 10 numerals are a standard way of representing numbers universally, although the symbols whereby these numbers are represented changes in certain cultures.

In modern computers all information is held as sequences of binary digits (0 or 1) or *bits*. Eight bits are considered to represent a computer "word" and are called a *Byte*. One Byte used to be the standard amount of data that was manipulated by a processor at any one moment in time, but many of the modern powerful processors work with "words" that are 16, 32 or more bits long. The characters of the alphabet are represented by internationally agreed codes and conventions. The most widely used scheme is ASCII (American Standard Code for Information Interchange), which uses 7 bits to provide 128 possible characters. An extended 8-bit ASCII covers 256 characters including the Greek alphabet. When ASCII is used for the underlying coding scheme for representing characters within a computer, sorted lists are presented in ASCII order. The numeric digits 0–9 precede the upper-case letters A–Z, which precede the lower-case letters a–z.

The limitations of ASCII are at once evident. Text has more features than just the characters: characters may be represented in many different "fonts" or styles and sizes, which alters their appearance and impact. And there are many more alphabets worldwide which have to be represented. In addition, text must be formatted for best effect, with indents, alignments, margins and so on. ASCII is unable to accommodate much of the current need for text representation. Further needs are for representation of mathematical and chemical formulae, graphics and many other specialised forms of data and information, which are completely beyond the scope of ASCII.

An important feature of computers is their ability to manipulate and communicate information in ways that are not possible with paper-based systems. Data may be recorded once and then used in different ways and places. This facility to reuse and communicate data is the key to delivering improvements in clerical and managerial productivity which have transformed other industries.

Computer systems

Every computer system comprises both hardware and software. The physical components of the system are known as *hardware*, while *software* refers to the computer programs which determine how the hardware can be used. An analogy with this book may help explain the difference. This book itself, its pages and cover, are equivalent to hardware, but software is the information it contains, represented by patterns of ink on pages.

Software can be divided up into three separate classes: the *operating system*, which sets up the computer and provides the housekeeping functions; the *applications* software, which contain the instructions for carrying out a specific set of functions, such as a word processor; and the **files** of text or data that are stored, processed and manipulated by the applications software on the computer.

The software in a computer cannot readily be perceived by the human observer, since it is held electronically, either as magnetic charges on disks or as electrical signals within the computer memory and processor chips. The electronic nature of the information held in a computer is the key to its easy access: the data can be accessed and used wherever there is a terminal that can link up to that computer across a network. Unlike a book, where a single copy can only be used by one person in one place at any moment in time, several people can look at the same information held on a computer at the same time and in different places.

Memory

Data is held in a computer as a series of bits, as outlined above. Eight (2^3) bits constitute a Byte; 1 kilobyte (KB) comprises 2^{10} or 1,024 Bytes; 1 megabyte (MB) comprises 2^{20} or 1,048,576 Bytes; 1 gigabyte (GB) comprises 2^{30} or 1,073,741,824 Bytes, and so on — the next larger unit is a terabyte (TB) which is 2^{40} or 1024 GB, and larger units will be designated as the need arises. Note that everything to do with computer memory is based on the binary system and powers of 2, which is why when you buy a 100MB disk, you may be surprised to find that you actually have nearly 105 million Bytes of data storage.

The bits are stored in memory. A memory device therefore has to have discrete locations, or *addresses*, where specific items of data are stored, and a means of representing two states, for the bits 0 and 1. Most widely used are magnetic media, where the states are represented by magnetic fields of opposite polarities. Because magnetism persists after it has been recorded (think of a cassette tape), data stored in this way is stable and durable, and can remain readable for a period of years. But the data can be easily erased by exposing the disk to a new magnetic field, so the disk can be reused and rerecorded at will, usually millions of times.

Magnetic disks come in "floppy" or "hard" forms: floppy disks are flexible, come in $3\frac{1}{2}$ or $5\frac{1}{4}$ inches diameter sizes, and are easily inserted and removed from disk drives which are normally mounted in the case of the computer; hard disks are usually mounted internally and are often referred to as "fixed". Some hard disks are removable, but these are expensive and generally used only for special purposes. However, new miniaturised removable hard disks are available for use with miniature "palm-top" computers and may become popular. A floppy disk typically stores in the region of 500 KB to 3 MB, whilst hard disks in current production typically store between 20 MB up to more than 1 GB. These numbers are continually increasing as technology progresses and storage densities increase. Magnetic tapes and tape cartridges (cassettes) are widely used as back-up media: the difference with tapes is that they are not "random access" as are disks, and the whole tape may have to be spooled through to find a specific block of data.

There are other durable storage media, such as optical media (think of your audio CD/compact disk), where the bits are stored as pits burned by a laser into a metal disk: these can be detected by another laser as variations in the reflection of light. CDs are mostly inerasable (called Write Once Read Many times or WORMs), and have an expected life of tens of years, although rewritable optical systems (e.g. magneto-optical disks (MOD)) are now available. Optical storage enables large amounts of data to be stored in a very compact form, typically about 600 MB on a normal audio compact disk (12 cm).

Various other memory and storage systems also exist (such as "bubble", magneto-optical etc.), most of which are not in widespread usage at the present time, although this is likely to change as needs and prices change. All storage media are "formatted", which means that sectors where data can be stored are defined and file allocation tables set up ready to receive the data. Different computer systems use different formats.

Chips

Data can also be stored in electronic chips, where it is represented as different voltages. The chips act as a bank of on/off switches (flip-flops), which turn on and off. When they are 'off', the voltage shown is zero, but when they are 'on' they link through to a higher voltage rail in the computer. This form of electronic data storage (mainly used as RAM — Random Access Memory) is not stable: when the power is switched off, the data is lost. However, they have the advantage that data stored in such chips can be accessed at very high speeds, typically in a few nanoseconds (10^{-9} seconds), making them ideal for temporary storage of data that is being processed by the computer.

However, there are forms of electronic storage which are stable when the power is switched off: these are called ROM, or Read Only Memory, devices because they are mostly designed to be used by the computer when it is "booting" up from the powered off state, when it reads its set-up information from these chips. ROM can be erased and reprogrammed using various techniques (called variously PROM, EPROM, EEPROM, depending on technology). These chips are widely used in smart cards, which need to hold data even when there is no power source attached.

Central Processor Unit (CPU)

The heart of every computer system is the *central processor unit*, normally a processor chip containing the equivalent of several million transistors. The power of a computer processor is related to the number of bits it can process at the same time (for example a 32-bit processor is normally more powerful than a 16-bit processor) and the number of computer **operations** or calculations that can be carried out in each second, usually expressed in MHz, or millions of calculation cycles (operations) per second.

However, these are not the only factors that determine the performance of a computer system. The CPU has a repertoire of operations that it can perform, called its instruction set: some CPUs have a complex instruction set, whilst others are simpler, or "reduced" (hence Reduced Instruction Set Computer — RISC). The instruction set determines the way in which a specific operation is performed, and the number of cycles that is required for that instruction to be executed.

The applications software instructs the system as to how to perform an operation, and this requires that specific pieces of data are retrieved from wherever they are stored and brought into memory locations where active processing by the CPU can take place, and then returned to storage elsewhere whilst another piece of data is processed. The movement of data around the computer, from disk storage to RAM storage, into registers (where processing takes place) and back is handled by the computer architecture and operating system. Speed and efficiency of data movements within the computer can exert a marked effect on overall performance.

The performance and speed of a system depends on its weakest link. Simplistic increases in processor speed, memory or disk capacity may well prove disappointing. However, removal of a bottleneck can sometimes produce a spectacular improvement for a small expenditure. In many systems the process of moving data onto and off the hard disk (input-output, or I/O) is a bottleneck. However a section of the RAM can be configured to act as a *cache*, to accept data that has been processed, and hold it until the I/O process is less busy: this can be especially effective in boosting system performance.

Expressing the performance of one computing system in terms that enable it to be compared with another is not easy, because of these variations. Various **benchmark** performance figures are quoted, based on the time taken to perform a set task, but the very nature of the task itself may favour one type of computer architecture over another. Alternative expressions are based on Millions of Instructions Per Second (MIPS), or Millions of FLoating point Operations Per Second (MFLOPS) for computations that are largely arithmetic in nature. Proprietary performance measurement systems also exist, but cannot generally be applied outside of the range of products from that manufacturer.

File-stores

All software is organised into **files.** Each file-store contains many files. Files are usually grouped together and placed in *directories*. A file-store contains one *root* directory only and this root directory may have any number of *subdirectories*, each of which may have further subdirectories and so on. Each directory may contain files, as well as subdirectories, but a file cannot contain any other file. Two files with identical names cannot exist in the same directory, but can co-exist in different directories in the same file-store.

Each directory is assigned a name: every directory has a direct linkage to the root directory. The entire store is organised into a tree structure (albeit inverted from the "normal" tree), where the directories are the branches, and the **files** are leaves of the tree For example see Figure 4.1.

A *path* can be described from any directory to any other. For example the path to FileF from the root goes through Sub1 and Sub11; the path from Sub2 to FileB goes through the Root and Sub1. Paths are used to tell the computer where to look for a file, and are written as sequential directions from the starting point to the destination, each step separated from the next by a specific symbol, usually a slash (/) or backslash (\). For example to tell the computer how to find FileF, one would describe the path from the root as: Sub1\Sub11\FileF.

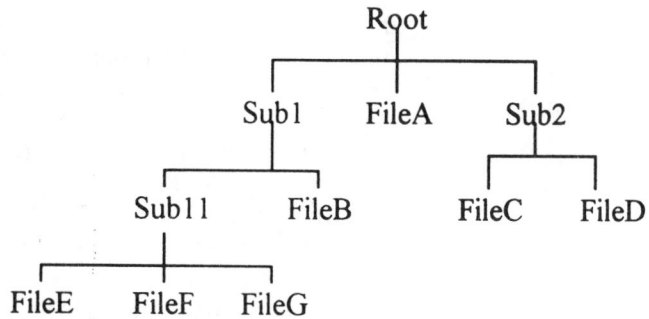

Figure 4.1

Files of a similar type are often stored in the same directory so that they can be found easily. There are many types of file, for programs, data and so on. To make it easier to know what is in a file, it is assigned a name, which should be meaningful at least to the person who named it, and usually an extension, which conventionally is used to indicate the type of file (e.g. word processed, database etc.). Therefore, for example "fred.doc" might be a word processed letter to Fred; "study.dbf" might be a database derived from a research study.

Data files may hold all manner of data, which may be coded, encrypted, and organised in any way appropriate to the applications software used to create the file. Thus most files are unreadable, except to one specific application.

In medical applications, many of the data files are derived from database applications. Database files, such as those used to compile patient registers, usually contain a number of different *records* each holding data about a different object or event (e.g. records of patients registered, or of care encounters). The information within each record is usually structured into *fields*. Each record has the same number of fields, and each field within a record contains data about the same feature or attribute of the object or event. For example the patient database might have fields for first name, last name, date of birth, sex etc.

Each field may contain data in different formats. The data may be recorded as a *string* of text (i.e. words) or *characters* (e.g. a code made up of letters, numbers and punctuation marks), or *numbers*, or it may record a *date* or a *logical* statement (true/false).

When files are "opened" for processing, the relevant piece of the file is brought from where it is stored on disk into RAM to make it more accessible for processing. Normally the file is closed, and returned to disk before the power is switched off. If this does not happen, the portions of the file held in RAM at the time of switching off will be destroyed. Hence there may be problems of data loss and corruption that arise when a computer system or its power supply fails.

Operating system

A computer cannot do anything without software. Software can be thought of as a set of layers. At the lowest level, directly controlling the hardware is the operating system. The operating system determines the character of the whole system: it determines what instructions can be recognised by the CPU, and is responsible for managing the various components of the system. Some of the software that controls the operations of the computer may be installed in the form of micro code or firmware that is loaded into ROM and is all but inseparable from the hardware itself. The same computer running a different operating system may seem quite different to the user.

For personal computers (PCs) the industry standard operating system is MS-DOS which only runs on the Intel range of micro-processors (e.g. Intel 80486). An enormous range of low cost applications software is available to run under MS-DOS. Various shells and presentation managers, such as Windows, can alter the "feel" of the system and provide added functionality on top of DOS. DOS can only run one process at a time (single tasking) and interact with one user, and has therefore never paid much attention to issues of file access security. However, the development of networking does much to overcome some of these limitations.

Larger computer installations which have multiple users and run multiple tasks simultaneously use a variety of operating systems. One of the most widely used is UNIX: UNIX was originally developed during the 1960s and is now available for a wide variety of platforms. As a multi-user system, it works efficiently even when many users are operating a variety of different terminals and using different applications at the same time. Each user is quite unaware that the computer's resources are being shared (time-sharing) with others. Additional users can be added by connecting further terminals or workstations at low cost. The security system controls access to files while record-locking prevents potential corruption of data when more than one person tries to modify a record at the same time.

Ports and peripherals

Most computers have a wide range of peripheral devices attached to them, using the *ports* or multi-pin plugs and sockets provided. The most commonly attached peripherals are a keyboard and monitor, and a printer. Many users would have a MODEM for communications.

Each peripheral device requires the data passing between it and the computer to conform to its own set of expectations. Thus the computer needs to know what each device attached to it is, so that the communications with it can be appropriately handled, and to which port that device is attached, so that it knows where to direct output to and expect input from. Each device generally requires a

41

driver to be loaded on the computer to manage this input-output data conversion.

Any mismatch between the speed at which the computer and a peripheral are able to handle data is handled by a *buffer* placed between the two devices: this is a small and temporary data store which can be filled quickly by the sender of information, and slowly emptied to the receiver (or vice versa).

Software applications

We are approaching the time when a personal workstation and corporate network is taken for granted as a basic office necessity, just as a desk and telephone are today. Soon most staff will have their own systems at home, and many will also have a palmtop in their pocket linked by radio to home and office networks. The issue will not be whether an institution can afford the cost of such systems but whether it can afford **not** to invest and thereby to risk losing competitive edge and staff.

Workstations and the user interface

Users' expectations are rising. Few are happy to revert to using a 'dumb' character-based terminal after using a colour graphics PC or workstation with a graphical user interface (GUI) using windows and icons. Windows refers to a style of computer screen display which allows the user to display overlapping frames, each containing a separate application. This permits fast and easy switching between multiple applications. MicroSoft-Windows is a *de facto* standard graphical user interface for PCs. Icons are graphical representations of objects, such as a file of information, or of tools used to do a task. For example, moving a file icon to a printer icon may cause the file to be printed. A mouse or similar pointing device is normally used to manipulate icons.

Workstations with graphical user interfaces (GUIs) are claimed to deliver significant benefits compared with dumb terminals. A well designed system leads to fewer operator errors, requires less training, improves user performance and confidence and gives greater job satisfaction. A skilled and happy workforce is a productive workforce.

For most users all they ever see of any computer is their own terminal or workstation, and printer. European Directive 90/270/EEC sets out environmental and ergonomic standards for employees who habitually use display screen equipment as a significant part of their work. Among other provisions it requires employers to install terminals and furniture that meet specified minimum standards including swivel/tilt display screen, separate tiltable keyboard, adequate working space and a seat with adjustable height and back rest. The use of ergonomically designed furniture is important, but so also is instruction in appropriate posture, and limitation of the maximum number of hours that a user may work per day and/or without a break at a computer terminal. Failure to observe these requirements may lead to liability for disabling injuries, such as tenosynovitis and back pain.

There are growing concerns about the possible health risk posed by electromagnetic radiation from cathode ray displays, and it seems inevitable that minimum standards for electromagnetic radiation and screening will shortly be specified.

Client-server architecture

Client-server computing splits the processing required by an application between two processors, the front-end (client) and the back-end (server). The front-end often runs on a personal computer that presents and manipulates data in a graphical easy-to-use, and intuitive way. This computer is connected by a network to larger file servers which are the "back-end" and are able to store and retrieve files and software applications for use by the front-end processors. The server may also take responsibility for data protection and various other functions on behalf of the entire system.

The client-server model is particularly suitable for enterprises, such as hospitals with large numbers of workstations and multiple applications. Client-server architecture enables integration of disparate systems, including mainframe or minicomputer legacy systems.

The client-server approach is economical. Networked personal computers and servers are able to take over tasks which had previously required larger and more expensive minicomputers and mainframes. The client-server approach exploits the processing power of both desktop and server machines. Other benefits claimed for the client-server approach include:

- Access to wide range of data from multiple servers by a single desktop PC
- Consistent user interface reduces training/learning time
- Integration with existing systems protects previous investment
- Client-server systems are scaleable — new servers and clients can be added as needs increase
- A number of different front-end applications may share the same back-end services (e.g. database) on the server
- Network administrators can readily control user access to sensitive data, trouble-shoot problems and alter desktop and server configurations
- Network traffic is greatly reduced by ensuring that only requested data is sent from server to PC for processing
- Where software applications are served from a file server to all users, software upgrades are readily undertaken for the whole organisation

Software criteria

Meyer[1] has identified ten general requirements which should be met by most software products, and could be used for evaluating any application.

1. **Correctness** — software products should perform their tasks exactly as defined by the requirements and specification
2. **Robustness** — software systems should function even in abnormal conditions
3. **Extendibility** — software products should be adaptable to external changes. Two principles are essential for ensuring extendibility. First, design simplicity; a simple architecture is always easier to adapt to changes than a complex one. Second, decentralisation; the more autonomous the modules in a software architecture, the higher the likelihood that a simple change affects just one module, or just a small number of modules, rather than triggering off a chain reaction over the whole system
4. **Reusability** — software products should be reusable, in whole or in part, for new applications
5. **Compatibility** — the ease with which software products may be combined with others
6. **Efficiency** — the software should make good and efficient use of hardware resources such as processors, internal and external memories, communication devices
7. **Portability** — software products may need to be transferred to other hardware and software environments (e.g. different processors or operating systems)
8. **Verifiability** — acceptance procedures, particularly test data, and procedures for detecting failures and tracing errors, should be easily prepared
9. **Integrity** — software systems should be able to protect their various components (programs, data, documents) against unauthorised access and modification
10. **Ease of use** — it should not be difficult for a user to learn the use of the software, how to operate it, prepare and input data, interpret the responses, recover from usage errors and so on

[1]Meyer (1988) *Object-Oriented Software Construction* Prentice Hall

General purpose applications

The average health professional is likely to use at least three types of application: word processor, spreadsheet and database. Each of these is explained briefly.

Word processors

Word processors are everywhere, and have now almost completely replaced the typewriter. All readers will have seen the output from a word processor, and most will have used one. This book was naturally written on a word processor. The advantages of word processors include:

- A document can be amended, altered, edited and reorganised with the minimum of effort
- The document can be previewed and displayed exactly as it will print
- As many "original" copies of a document can be made as required
- The document can be sent electronically and instantly as a file to anywhere in the world
- The material is searchable, so that spelling and grammar errors can be detected, contents lists and indexes can be created automatically etc.
- Different character styles, fonts and sizes, and symbols can be intermixed, providing much greater flexibility in preparation of copy
- Pictures and tables can be created and embedded in the text, and the text laid out around them

In essence, all word processors work in the same way, although each of them uses different keystrokes to achieve the same result, and most have developed their own ways of representing characters internally in the computer. Each character (for example the letter 'a' or 'A') is encoded in digital form. These characters are displayed and manipulated according to sets of rules incorporated in the application, together with additional instructions, for example relating to formatting, character font and size that the user assigns. The end result may be displayed on screen, printed, or sent electronically to another location.

One issue that quite often confuses users is that a word processor views every character, including a space or a line feed (or "carriage return" as it is still often called) instruction as a discrete entity which can therefore be edited, moved and deleted like any other character. Spaces are not voids to the word processor. Many word processors have an option which enables you to display every entity, including formatting and font instructions, on screen.

Spreadsheets

The spreadsheet is one of the most widely used computer applications, perhaps because there are so many ways in which it can contribute to the efficient management of, especially numerical, data. The purpose of the spreadsheet is the manipulation of numbers, and the calculation of repetitive formulae: one of the most important uses of spreadsheets, therefore, is in managing finances and providing for the accounting needs of individuals and businesses. However, it also has wide application in simple statistics, and in displaying numeric data in a variety of graphical representations that enhance the meaning and impact of the data.

Basic spreadsheet features

The spreadsheet consists of columns and rows. The rows are assigned a "name" in the form of a number from 1 up to a maximum defined by the software (but usually more than 1000 rows are permitted in any single spreadsheet file). The columns are named using characters from A–Z, then from AA–AZ, then BA–BZ and so on, again up to the maximum permitted by the software (usually in the region of 500 or so columns).

At the intersection of a column (e.g. B) and a row (e.g. 2) there is a cell (B2): every cell in the spreadsheet is named according to the column and row which intersect upon it. Thus the general format of a spreadsheet is as below:

COLUMNS

		A	B	C	D	E	F	G
	1	A1	B1	C1	D1	E1	F1	G1
	2	A2	B2	C2	D2	E2	F2	G2
R	3	A3	B3	C3	D3	E3	F3	G3
O	4	A4	B4	C4	D4	E4	F4	G4
W	5	A5	B5	C5	D5	E5	F5	G5
S	6	A6	B6	C6	D6	E6	F6	G6
	7	A7	B7	C7	D7	E7	F7	G7

A CELL may contain:

- Characters (e.g. a text header or note)
- Numbers
- Formula
- Date
- Other (such as logical statements, true/false etc.)

Formulae in spreadsheets

The essential functionality of a spreadsheet is conferred by the capacity to hold formulae in a cell. Normally the formulae within a cell are hidden from view (although software switches can be set to display formulae). The display relating to each cell is the *product* of the computation that is specified by the formula it holds. For example if the formula in a cell (say cell B3) instructs the computer to take the number displayed in another cell (say cell B2, which displays the number '2.6') and multiply it by 7, then the cell B3 will show the number 18.2 (2.6*7). However the real "contents" of cell B3 is a formula which is of the form:

$$B3 = B2*7$$

Note the use of the common mathematical symbol * to represent multiplication

Consequently the display in cell B3 is not fixed: it varies depending upon the number displayed by cell B2. If B2 is altered such that it now displays the number 1.2, B3 changes automatically to display a new number 8.4 (1.2*7), still true to the formula in that cell.

Any combination of the following functions, and often others, can be used in formulae:

Operations: Add(+), Subtract(−), Multiply(*), Divide(/),

Functions: Exponential, Logarithm Sum, Average,

Maximum, Minimum, Standard Deviation

Logical Statements:
Is equal to(=), is not equal to is less than(<), is greater than(>)

And Not Or

Use

Raw numerical data is entered into the spreadsheet as a set of numbers in specific assigned cells. The spreadsheet is set up (programmed) by the user to display derivatives of these numbers according to the formulae in the cells. The products of these calculations are displayed in the spreadsheet and constitute information. Spreadsheets are ideal for:

- Providing up-to-date information on financial position
- Deriving information from raw data by application of fixed formulae
- Predicting the consequences of contingencies ("what . . . . if . . .")

There is almost no limit to the complexity of the formulae, or of the derived data structures that can be created within a spreadsheet. The formulae effectively link cells together, but there is no need for linked cells to have any physical proximity to one another. Indeed, if you decide to rearrange your spreadsheet by moving blocks of cells around using the editing functions, which are essentially exactly the same as in the word processor, (i.e. Move, Copy, Delete etc.), the linkages between cells are maintained, even though the physical locations may have been changed.

Spreadsheets have a range of reporting tools, including graphic displays. Thus data may be put into a spreadsheet just in order to display it as a graph, bar chart or "pie" chart. Data displays are especially important in converting tables of data, which may not be readily understood by the reader, into graphical information, which is readily appreciated and understood.

Databases

Databases are used for tracking and finding objects, and for organising and sorting records about those objects in flexible ways.

A database consists of records: each record normally relates to one object or event, and is composed of a number of fields. Each field of the record describes a specific attribute of the object, and that same field in successive records describes that same attribute of successive objects. Each field may contain numbers, dates, logic (True/False) or characters (which may include numbers as well as text). Each field has a defined length in most databases: a specified number of bytes, or spaces, are assigned to that field, and that sets the maximum number of characters the field can hold. If the field turns out to be too small, the structure of the whole database has to be altered to increase the size of that field in every record of the database.

The purpose of a database is for organising and sorting records, for example to find records that match a description, or to find all those which share one or more features in common, or to arrange a large number of records in a specified order (e.g. alphabetic). Patient master indexes, research and analysis systems, clinical records and laboratory systems are all typically built around a database engine. Lists of names and addresses, for example, of suppliers, patients or providers are typically held in a database. These lists can be sorted to identify, for example, all patients due for immunisation, or for cervical screening, and those records extracted can be merged with a standard letter to create a personalised recall: a set of sticky name and address labels can be printed at the same time to reduce the time required for addressing.

For example, a small research database into blood pressures might contain records about a group of patients using the following fields:

Surname

First name

Sex

Age

Systolic (blood pressure)

Diastolic (blood pressure)

Heart Rate

and look something like:

	Surname	First Name	Sex	Age	Systolic	Diastolic	Heart Rate
1	Warner	Adrian	M	3	107	78	135
2	Peterson	Mary	F	3	108	81	145
3	Wurth	Janine	F	6	115	79	120
4	Tomlinson	Thomas	M	41	155	95	85

etc.

A database is similar to a card index: both record attributes of separate objects or events. Both require that the attributes are recorded once only. The fundamental difference is that whilst a card index can only be arranged in one order, an electronic database can be arranged into as many different orders as may be useful to their users. The same database can be reordered (sorted) electronically into any primary and secondary order of attributes that is requested by users without any disruption of its basic structure. It can also be used to find objects that fit specific search patterns or specified attributes.

To make best use of such a system it is essential to know what data is recorded and how that data is classified and organised. The structure of a database identifies the fields that it contains, as well as the length and type of each field. A field can be of almost any length: however, the shorter it is the faster the database can be manipulated. Thus short fields are preferable, and hence concise coded entries are preferable where feasible over free text.

Chapter 5　Planning and procuring a system

Management of change

Successful implementation of any computer system requires careful planning. The secret is not so much in doing things right, since there are many ways to achieve the goal, but in avoiding those pitfalls that have already been identified as well trodden pathways towards disaster. **Technology** is not usually the major problem — in most instances it is not a problem at all. The real risks in a project are nearly all related to **people**. Poorly designed software can often be highly successful when implemented with the support, understanding and co-operation of the people: on the other hand the best system in the world can prove a disaster if it lacks that support.

Planning the introduction of any computer system is a politically charged process. It will change the way that many people do their work and the distribution of power within the organisation. Remember that information gives power. Many of those within an organisation who are now in power have achieved their positions through their ability to make the "old" order work for them, and through accumulating experience in the field. The advent of technology poses two clear threats to these people: first the ways of doing things will change, and new skills and expertise will be required; second under the proposed "new" order a relative newcomer will be able to call upon information that they may have spent years in accumulating and have a vested interest in keeping to themselves.

Support and champions

Machiavelli recognised the precarious nature of the role of an agent of change. Any change is likely to encounter the entrenched opposition of the existing holders of power. At best, support for it will be lukewarm and will come from those who perceive that they might improve their status under the new order. These supporters will soon disappear if at any stage the project falters.

Every project needs support at two levels. There must be high level support from the chief executive, which unequivocally creates an expectation of change for the organisation. In addition there must be support from those who are to be affected by the proposed changes at the workface. The Project Board that is selected to manage the project must reflect this, with members elected or selected so as to ensure the full backing and support of general management, information systems staff, clinicians and nurses.

The project needs a champion who can sell a realistic view of the future when the system has been successfully implemented. However, it is important also not to "oversell" the benefits, since this may lead users to expect too much too soon. The full benefits of any new system may take months or even years to accrue, not weeks. In many instances the benefits will, in part, depend on the external environment, for example the rate of penetration of systems, and the speed of take-up of EDI in the region.

The process of enlisting the support of the various strategic groups must start from the earliest possible moment. It is difficult to conceal that a change is in the wind. When this leaks out, people are inclined toward pessimism and suspect the worst in terms of the impact on themselves. In the absence of clear indications or intentions, rumours sweep the workplace, and before you know it the staff will be opposed to the plan even though they have no idea what it is they are opposing.

Winning the support of these groups is best done in face-to-face meetings and open discussions, and not just through formal presentations. Such interactive meetings are a two-way learning process for both the project manager and the users, during which objections, reservations, fears and worries should be brought out, and support and confidence in the proposal can be developed.

Management of change

Change is a relatively slow process. Even with a positive attitude to the change, people who are affected by the change will take time to understand it, learn new skills and to internalise the use of the new system as a part of their everyday routines.

Change creates uncertainty: where there is uncertainty there is fear and rumour. The management of this requires investment of time and effort, and the use of appropriate ways to involve those who will be affected by it. This requires support and active listening, and the use of tools such as workshops, seminars, consultations sessions and newsletters to gain their commitment and involvement.

Staff must be motivated by management to view the change as positive and beneficial and to become committed to it. They must embrace the goals of the change and be prepared to work towards their achievement. In addition there will need to be serious investment in appropriate education and staff development activities.

Expectations of change are frequently unrealistic, both high and low of the mark. Their expectations determine whether staff will be pleased with the outcomes of the change. Expectation management should be a key element of the change management process. The goal must be to deliver slightly more and to deliver it slightly sooner than is generally expected, and sooner than has been promised.

Expectation management

Management of expectations from highest to lowest level within an organisation is a key element of management of the change, and is frequently a source of difficulty. IT developments frequently evoke unrealistic expectations, both high (from those who believe in IT wizardry) and low (from those who are eternally cynical). IT remains poorly understood by the majority. Clear and concise information must be provided regularly and frequently throughout the process to ensure expectations are realistic. Delivery should always be planned to be slightly better than that promised in terms of timing and cost. There is little that is technically impossible in the world of IT: the goal is to select or develop that which is practical, beneficial, easy to use and cost-effective.

Vendors frequently have to sell based on promises of applications yet to be developed, or "vapourware" as it is often called. They are not entirely to blame for this, since purchasers often pursue unrealistic dreams and press for impossible terms and conditions, which must be agreed to in order to secure the business. Failure to secure business means that it will go to a competitor who, in all probability, is also selling vapourware and is at least as unlikely to deliver on promises on time and on budget. Realism needs to prevail. There will always be predictions of what could and should be available soon. Visits to reference sites involve reviewing the operation of products that may be stable, but are probably obsolete, especially beneath the surface veneer. It is important to evaluate vendor claims with independent and confidential informatics advice.

Procurement

Procuring and implementing a computer system is analogous to setting out on a long voyage. It pays handsomely to plan ahead, to consult widely, to prepare plans for likely contingencies, and to consider all of the foreseeable consequences. From the outset, you will have access to a mass of information and advice from suppliers, who probably want to sell you their wares, and from colleagues who may have undertaken similar journeys in the past. Most of the advice you receive will be sound and well-meaning, but every situation is different, and your final decisions must be based on your specific needs.

An enormous amount of scarce healthcare computing expertise is devoted to procurement of computer systems with doubtful benefits. The most obvious mistakes made repeatedly by hospitals come, not from selecting the wrong supplier, but from failure to resource adequately the management of change, implementation and training.

Tender and procurement costs

The cost of the procurement exercise can easily exceed 30 per cent of the total cost of a system. The purchaser produces a voluminous specification, typically in excess of 100 pages for a significant system: the potential suppliers have learned to play safe by responding with similarly voluminous but essentially standard word-processed responses to requests for proposals (RFPs). Indeed many suppliers refrain from tendering unless they can use an off-the-shelf proposal virtually unchanged.

Sadly, the approach that is so often adopted appears to be driven more by a desire to prove breach of contract by the supplier than by any expectation that it could lead to a successful implementation. The outcome that seems to be anticipated from the way this process is conducted is one of disputation. It seems to be expected that there will be a withholding of due payments and/or litigation based on some elements of the specification or vendors proposal. With this as an up-front expectation, there is every probability that it will happen, and further expenses will be incurred all round.

Few purchasers know exactly what it is they want at the time when they are trying to specify it. Fewer still have knowledge of all the various solutions that have been developed to address this issue, nor of how they have been conceptualised and modelled, and very few have an adequate knowledge of relevant information technology trends and developments. As a consequence the specification is often unduly restrictive: it may even expressly require adoption of inappropriate or obsolete technologies in order to meet certain clauses (the authors recall one recent tender which required a punched card reader facility, even though these belong to the distant past of computing). By the time the product is delivered, the knowledge, understanding and requirements of the purchaser will have moved on: a process of reinterpretation of the specifications and undertakings given then ensues in an attempt by both sides to move the goalposts.

Supplier and purchaser need to *share* their knowledge and understanding in the development of an acceptable solution. A partnership is likely to be more productive than an adversarial relationship together with an approach to development based on fast prototyping, where various ways of achieving the goal may be tried out in "draft" form and progressively refined to see which best meets the real needs of the users.

But far more important is the issue of the future, of taking into account the changes in user needs and technology that must happen — in other words the whole issue of "future-proofing" of the acquisition. It is generally impossible to predict the future, although some clear trends can be identified. It is difficult, but not impossible, to develop a solution that can accommodate change. For example, a solution that is developed based on a well researched model of the environment being computerised, using object-oriented techniques, modular rather than monolithic, and created using fourth generation programming languages (4GLs) is likely to be readily modifiable and remain serviceable for a relatively long time.

Project management

A project manager should be appointed, responsible to the project board. He or she will need energy to push changes through, enthusiasm to learn as much as possible about how the system can be used, and a vision of what life will be like when the system is fully implemented.

The first priority is to sell the idea to prospective users. The identification of a local "champion" is invaluable: he or she can take the lead role in promoting the plan to colleagues. It is important to ensure that users' expectations are kept in line with reality, to focus attention on existing, recognised problems, and to stimulate concern that something has to be done now to tackle these problems. It helps if there is already a general expectation that changes are inevitable.

The project manager needs to decide the tactics for the system's introduction, what functions are to be used first by which users, and how the system will meet the specified needs. These matters require a high level of knowledge and practical understanding of healthcare computing, of how the current and proposed systems work, and of the personalities involved.

Regular progress reviews are required to check that each step is completed according to plan, that manual systems are discontinued, and that everyone is doing what was expected of them. This helps to identify bottlenecks and slippages so that action can be taken before they threaten the entire project.

It is greatly encouraging to evaluate the benefits and tell people what progress has been made, so that they can see and recognise their own shared achievements. This builds morale and maintains motivation, as well as providing a baseline for planning and justifying further developments.

Training requires a dedicated facility in a quiet location with minimal risk of disturbance from telephones or bleeps. Staff being trained must fully allocate their time to training and make arrangements to cover their normal duties. Training is a big job in itself; installing a maternity system in one hospital required organising nearly 100 sessions to train 300 midwives, clerical staff and other users.

Each new procedure needs to be documented, job descriptions edited and new staff training and induction programmes modified accordingly.

Developing your own solution

In practice the purchaser finds himself confronted by making a choice between a limited number of fairly standard solutions, or developing something to fit the needs identified. In all probability one or more off-the-shelf solutions will be identified that can provide 60–80 per cent of what is required. There is a choice of whether to adopt and adapt one of these, to modify the requirements to fit one of the available products, or to enter into a new development.

The urge to develop an entirely new solution must be strong, given the large numbers of people who choose that route. However, the costs of such a project are high and the chances of recouping those costs based on the development of a commercially viable product that is resold to other users is rather small. Furthermore the work entailed in supporting, maintaining and continuing the development of a one-off product is high. Unless all these issues have been carefully weighed up, it is probably not the best way to go. Software engineering is not a job for enthusiastic amateurs.

Adapting a product that meets most but not all of the requirements may be successful and produce an acceptable solution. For this to be viable, it is important that the product is engineered in a flexible environment that is amenable to the required changes. It is also worth remembering that the new features are likely to require a considerable amount of "tweaking" before they are just what the users want, which will make the project larger than may have been anticipated. This is often approached by forming a joint venture between developer and client, with a view to commercial marketing of the modified applications, using the location where the development is undertaken as a reference site. Whatever the arrangements that are made, it is important that there is adequate resourcing for the project to be completed: in most instances the client should also have in-house software engineering capabilities and access to the source code of the applications.

Costing your acquisition

The costs of your system are made up principally of:

non-recurrent:
- Hardware
- Software purchase, licenses, adaptation
- Communications, interfaces and networks
- Security and provision for disaster recovery

recurrent

- Maintenance and IT support (typically 10–15 per cent of purchase price)
- Communication costs (where third party networks are used).
- Education, training and user support

As time goes by your system will become out-of-date, both in terms of what it does and of the hardware that it uses to do it. It will need a major overhaul or even total renewal every so often. However, at the same time the cost of hardware is falling and the performance of software is improving, which means that in 2 years time you could replace your whole system for perhaps 30–60 per cent of the original cost. But of course by then everyone has decided that they need more memory, power and performance. Many institutions are faced with the realisation that the mainframe system they bought 5 years ago and invested in heavily is now becoming hopelessly expensive to maintain, and could better be replaced by a network of PCs. Downsizing of the central processors is becoming a business imperative.

Legacy systems

Many procurements are made more complicated as a consequence of previous investments in systems. In most instances the development cannot take place in a "green field" because there are numerous legacy systems remaining in place: these may carry out their niche tasks well, but almost all of them are likely to be representatives of earlier technologies.

The costs of trying to incorporate legacy systems into the final solution may be excessive, in terms of interfacing and networking. The constraints they may impose on the decisions to be taken may be counter-productive. It is often wiser to consider excluding legacy systems, either by scrapping them, or by allowing them to continue operating outside the "new" environment until due for replacement, which can be seen as the next phase of the overall information systems plan development.

Sources of funding

Information systems will continue to be a major capital expenditure item. So what options are there for funding? There is no single solution, but institutions may care to consider at least some of the following.

You could **buy.** If you buy, you own the equipment, can depreciate it and you have no recurrent financing charges. However it does make a major hole in your capital budget, and commits you to a specific collection of hardware components which will grow obsolete and will break down in time.

You could consider commercial **hire purchase,** where you would borrow the required funds. Once again you own the equipment and can depreciate it, but have the same disadvantages of obsolescence and deterioration. The interest on your borrowings may be tax deductible, but the availability of finance and its cost is not always predictable.

You might consider a **finance lease,** where you are obligated to purchase the equipment at the end of the agreed period for an agreed residual value. This may have special benefits, such as that 100 per cent of the value can be financed so eliminating any need for capital budgetary provision. The lease is normally at fixed interest, so provision for payments is predictable even though commercial interest rates may vary. The lease may be able to be revised to include equipment upgrades or additions. The equipment normally becomes yours at the end of the lease, which means that you carry the benefits/risks of ownership: however the lessor does not have to sell you the equipment at the agreed residual price so you may be accepting some risks without the benefits. Careful negotiation of the residual can defray this risk. There may be provisions required for disclosure of such leases in a statement of accounts. In addition lease payments are a commitment that must be serviced.

You could think of an **operating lease.** These differ from the above in that there is no obligation to purchase at the end of the lease, and that leased equipment may be upgraded and updated after an agreed period of usage. There may also under some circumstances be balance sheet disclosure advantages to these leases, and future payments need not be shown as a future liability. However, you do not own the equipment.

Finally there are **rentals.** Rentals tend to be shorter term, typically 1–2 years, but have most of the characteristics of an operating lease. They are generally only useful where you wish to have equipment only for a short time, or perhaps wish to try it out before deciding on whether to organise some other longer term funding arrangement.

Benefits realisation

The benefits of information systems do not just happen. They must be identified, quantified (where possible) with realistic agreed targets, and then realisation must be planned and monitored. Each hospital contemplating a major IT project should establish a formal Benefits Project covering investment appraisal and benefits realisation. The Benefits Project should result in:

1. Staff committed to success of investment and willing to work for benefits identified
2. The current performance of the unit will be closely examined. The potential benefits, whether cash-releasing or qualitative, will be identified, quantified and targets set
3. Alternative options should be set out. The options considered should cover a wide range including "doing nothing", "wheelbarrow" and "Rolls-Royce" options, with their relative costs and benefits
4. A plan for realisation of benefits, specifying who is responsible, when benefits are to be achieved and what resources will be made available. This plan provides a framework for the post-implementation review

Action teams

Large projects can be subdivided and small Action Teams set up for each area of impact. If a project involves several directorates, then each directorate should set up its own action team. Each team should include representatives from both clinical and business areas, and, once a supplier has been chosen, a supplier representative. (Make sure to budget for the time needed.)

Staff savings

Staff savings are an obvious way of justifying the cost of the computer system, but no one likes to make loyal staff compulsorily redundant. There are other ways of realising manpower savings:

- Natural wastage
- Early retirement
- Overtime reduction
- Staff redeployment
- Change of skill mix or grades needed
- Change from full time to part time
- Reduction in agency staff
- Increased productivity and throughput

User support

Support by IT professionals is essential. There must be a help desk, which provides a single point of contact for all types of problems. An unhelpful or unavailable help desk is a sure way to alienate the user community. IT staff have to see the system users as clients of their service rather than problems to be avoided or ignored. This has to be supported by technical staff with knowledge and skills sufficient to manage hardware and software problem analysis and management. It is unlikely that an in-house electronic engineering facility will be able to compete in terms of cost or time for hardware repairs, and this sort of service might well be considered for outsourcing.

Some practical suggestions and hints

Preparation

Key staff must be involved as early as possible in the development and implementation of IT plans. A champion must be found. Visits to vendor reference sites are vital as a means of managing expectations through personal evaluation of the impact of the system on normal staff activities. When a system has been selected, some time spent by key staff learning its use at a working site will be a worthwhile investment.

The starting point — look forwards

Many organisations, large and small, are daunted by the task of loading vast amounts of data from previous years, often from paper records, onto the new system. This may not be necessary: most information has a relatively rapid decay time and is no longer useful. The day the new computer system starts up should be seen as day one of a new era. All future information will be committed to computer, but past information will mostly remain where it is. The two information systems, old and new, will run side by side for a short period, and any vital information that is still relevant can be transferred in summary only as and when it is identified — for example when that patient next attends for an appointment. Typically within less than 12 months the old system can become an archive.

Incremental or big bang?

Most systems can be introduced incrementally, for example, one function or module at a time, and in one department or unit at a time. This provides for operational experience, and a higher ratio of support staff to users. Managed carefully this can enhance the reputation of the product and make the next stages of implementation much easier. There are instances where simultaneous introduction of the same modules into two units can be valuable, creating a competition between them at individual and unit level as to the quickest and best implementation.

Self-help

Development of adequate user support facilities is manpower intensive. Self-help groups can reduce the pressure on IT professionals. Staff from the same areas of an institution can be formed into effective self-help groups by bringing them together for education and training at the same time: they will then naturally tend to look to each other first for help with difficulties before calling the help desk. Another useful plan has been the formation of "computing first aid" stations, where one or more individuals (generally from the secretarial or technical staff) normally working in a stable location and with a good knowledge of specific software applications are trained to cope with the most common user problems. This concept has proven valuable in improving the accessibility of first level support, and reducing the load on the IT professional staff.

Information and newsletters

A regular newsletter which reports on developments and achievements can be invaluable in boosting morale and the sense of achievement. Including material on current topics of interest and useful user hints can also provide an important educational tool. A small publication produced frequently is more effective than one that is large but infrequently produced.

Learning in one's own time

Getting the right people to attend sessions always presents problems. Long experience shows that senior staff, and especially clinical staff, simply do not attend as scheduled. One can organise individual tutorials, and in some instances that may be necessary. Development of a course that individuals can follow in their own time and at their own pace is invaluable. Putting the course onto a PC that they can take away and use in the privacy of their own office or home is even better. Training facilities should be open to users for extended hours, and preferably 24 hours a day, as long as that does not cause problems with security. Setting up courseware that is available on-line throughout the institution can help.

Information services (IS)

Typically, information services staff are unknown and unseen by the rest of the institution. Often that is because there are so many unhappy users! The isolation of the IS unit does nothing to help them recognise or resolve whatever problems there may or may not be. In implementing a system, IS staff must be customer focused salespeople, visiting and listening to their clients and ensuring their satisfaction. Personal contacts with the clients and gaining a better understanding of their business is as important a role for IS staff as technical and operational performance. Taking steps to ensure that back-ups and other times of system non-availability are well publicised and do not interfere with important activities is just one example of that customer focus. Being highly visible, prepared and articulate is important: joining in general and social activities is also invaluable.

Recognition

The process of information system development is one of learning new concepts and acquiring new skills. Often management, who may be in large part insulated from this effort, fails to appreciate it or to recognise the value of these skills to the organisation. The value can be looked at in terms of organisations productivity and performance improvements. The investment in people can also be viewed in a very pragmatic way: there is a cost in terms of time and effort involved in training a new recruit to become a productive member of staff. The investment (from both sides) in people must be recognised and valued.

Assurance

Many developments depend for their success on the presence and skills of a small number of key players: absence of any one of them, for whatever reason, could put the project at risk. Ensuring that their skills are understudied and their system-specific knowledge is fully documented is vital to assure the continuity of the project.

Single point of contact

Any relationship, whether between vendor and purchaser, or IS and clients, needs integrity. The authors have seen too many implementations become confused and delayed because too many individuals on both sides tried to get involved. The provider of services should ensure that they identify their client. In the case of a system purchase, there should be a designated account manager at the supplier end, liaising with an identified project manager at the purchaser end. All communications should flow through or be copied to these individuals. The same applies between information services and departments of the institution. Integrity of these relationships is vital for success.

System flexibility and growth

No information system is ever complete: it will be in a continual state of development. New modules will be acquired, older applications will be modified or discarded, new links will be conceived, and existing databases will need to be expanded to accommodate new information. Recognition of this at an early stage suggests certain requirements of the basic design of the system you acquire.

The ability of the software modules to inter-work will depend upon their adherence to certain standards both for representation of information (classification and coding) and for communications and interconnection. Where manufacturers have used higher level programming languages in the development of the software (e.g. Fourth Generation languages or 4GLs) there is often a greater prospect of being able to develop and modify the software quickly and cost-effectively than where older languages have been used. However, much will still depend upon the way in which the software was conceived by its designer.

Over time your system will grow and change. As your system grows it will probably require a more powerful platform, and this may mean new operating systems and software. Probably the only thing that you will want to take with you is the data you have collected. The value of the data stored within a system normally far exceeds the value of the system itself. However the data may have been stored in a form (e.g. coded, encrypted) that makes it difficult to extract and/or translate into a form suitable for loading into another system: careful attention to data file structures is important.

Proprietary versus open

Manufacturers of systems have in many instances solved computing problems in their own unique ways — hence the proliferation of operating systems, communications environments and so on. Each of these has been developed to meet a need, has been expensive to develop and so is guarded as commercial property, and probably protected by patent or copyright. Proprietary environments have been used in many instances to lock customers into buying from a specific vendor: the industry recognises that once a purchaser has been hooked by such a system, the chances of them going elsewhere for additional resources are very small. The reasons for this are that:

- They will have to junk most if not all of their existing proprietary resources
- They will probably be unable to convert much of their data stored in proprietary ways
- They cannot go to another vendor for modules since the technology they are using is exclusive

Adoption of proprietary systems not only locks users into a specific vendor, but also frequently locks them out of access to new technology which that vendor does not or cannot support.

The growing need to communicate between systems has led to the development of a new approach to the issue: the concept is that of "open systems". Any vendor can supply parts of the system and supply enhancements and developments, so fostering competitive pricing and increasing the number of groups developing value added services and features for open systems.

Despite the inherent sense in the adoption of the open systems concept, the enormous commercial investment in proprietary environments is a powerful source of self-interest. Many vendors have built interfaces between the more common proprietary systems thereby in part achieving a similar, if less elegant, solution to the connectivity problem.

The future for timely and cost-effective systems development lies in widespread adoption of standards, so that applications and modules can simply be plugged in and will run and communicate without further major investment of time or resources by the purchaser.

Island-thinking

A frequent area of misjudgment relates to the extent to which your information system can exist as an island of information. In reality it cannot: the value of an information system is largely a function of its ability to link with other modules and systems, local and remote, large and small. In fact your "system" is itself likely to be a large number of linked systems, each of which fulfills one element of your overall needs, and each of which must share some or all of its data with others.

Island thinking has led many institutions into a search for the ultimate "integrated" system: this has now largely been abandoned since, even were these available off the shelf, their monolithic structure would make them unable readily to be adapted and developed. Current developments are based on "interfaced" or "connected" systems, where the emphasis is on defining the interfaces between the systems and ensuring that all modules can be made to conform to these interface definitions. This has led to an increased demand for and emphasis on the development of standards.

IT policy

Institutional investment in information technology is growing rapidly, although not always in a co-ordinated way. Some of the IT investment may arise out of major IS projects, but a variable (and sometimes substantial) proportion may be driven by the various units in the organisation based on their own perceived priorities and using their own resources. Because institutional resources to support and maintain IT are limited, the cost-effectiveness and sustainability of these developments are of serious concern. These considerations should (but often do not) cause an overall IT policy to be developed.

Standardisation at a local level is essential if the institution is to achieve optimal benefit from its investment, and the initiative is to be sustainable. Setting appropriate local standards is important because, for example:

- Where the range of computing platforms and software supported is restricted, fewer information services staff will be required to install, support and maintain them because they are all essentially the same
- Restricting the range of platforms reduces the problems of interfacing between different systems
- Ensuring that all workstations use the same version of each software package reduces the need for support training, since there will be expert users in every area of the institution: all that is required is identification of local experts, and encouragement to use them
- Where the same software and systems are available at every workstation, staff can comfortably move (e.g. when transferred, promoted, covering someone off sick) without needing to re-learn: it is only necessary to invest time and resources in learning the system once for each staff person

Since the very early days of microcomputers it has been apparent that the diversity of hardware and software offerings in the market-place have had the potential to create problems regarding technical support, user education and training, and data interchange. Many of these problems persist today despite the development of a range of interface products and promulgation of Open Systems Interconnection protocols.

One issue of special concern relates to the burgeoning use of PCs and PC networks. These are widely used by units or individuals and may be operated as independent systems. Nevertheless they may store information which is of vital concern to the institution and often to the patients too. Ensuring that these systems conform with the general policies of the organisation in relation to privacy, security, data integrity and operational availability presents a problem. They often use software that has been developed by an enthusiastic amateur but has not been subjected to any sort of quality assurance of fitness for the purpose. They may operate without any attention to security or backing up of data, and be exchanging private and confidential information with other systems over links that are intrinsically insecure. They may be used to make and communicate decisions and orders without any thought given to the need for audit trails and legal evidence requirements. This is an issue of growing importance for effective management by information services personnel.

Institutional IT policy must cover the development of an integrated approach to systems as well as effective management of privacy concerns.

Bases of opposition to IT policy

The development of policy, formal or informal, of the type outlined above may be resisted by staff for many reasons, prominent amongst which are:

1. Personal efficiency — users familiar with one IT product or environment are unwilling to learn another. [This same issue arises when a recommended institutional "standard" (e.g. for a word processor package) has to be replaced as a consequence of political or technical developments.]
2. Personal freedom — users may wish not to conform, occasionally (but not often in the authors' experience) for good reasons such as technical or functional limitations, or a desire to experiment; many clinical units have access to finances whose expenditure is not subject to institutional policy and they can thereby circumvent any formal impediments to purchase
3. Suspicion — IT users may be unconvinced of the purity of the motives behind moves towards standardisation, or of the expertise of those involved in the promulgation of standards, and may react against them
4. Competition — departments of an institution are in continual competition for status often to the detriment of the functionality of the institution as a whole: this has been referred to above. IT may figure significantly in this equation, because competition for

status often wastes resources through acquisition of grandiose IT installations and/or use of non-standard software

5. Social and Political concerns — various "political" positions may be infringed by moves towards IT development and standardisation, prominent amongst which are:
    - Concerns about data security and possible misuse of information when a networked environment is created
    - Concerns about degradation of personal status and power; where information is power, any information system developments are likely to prove threatening to some senior decision-makers.
    - Feelings of guilt and personal inadequacy; individuals with limited knowledge of IT frequently attempt to sabotage IT developments to defer their need to address the problem.

Of course there are many good reasons for opposing restrictive policies, such as the need to comply with standards from elsewhere (for example where units from different institutions are involved in a common study) and the fact that there are genuine strengths and weaknesses of every platform and software package.

Insourcing and outsourcing IT services

The concept of "outsourcing" is that a service or set of services is purchased from a second organisation and makes use of personnel who are not employees of the first organisation. For example, the use of contract and agency staff are examples of outsourcing of a service.

The Information Services that typically might be considered for outsourcing are:

- Consultancy services
- Staff
- Software development and maintenance
- Operational systems management (facility management, FM)
- Education and training services

In some major development projects it may be desirable to consider outsourcing responsibility for what is now termed *systems integration* (SI). SI embraces a range of services, usually including:

- Prime contractor for a project comprising several companies and products
- Project monitoring and ensuring that all activities are co-ordinated and delivered on time
- Risk management and accepting responsibility for ensuring that there is no derailment of the development for whatever reason
- Quality management and implementation of a quality system to detect inconsistencies, errors and misalignment of components of the overall plan

- Contract management, ensuring that all contractors involved in the project deliver agreed services and equipment as required
- Technical integration, ensuring that the equipment is functionally interfaced, including interworking with legacy systems
- Migration planning, ensuring that there is a smooth transition from old to new environments
- Staff development, ensuring that staff are prepared to work effectively and efficiently within the new environment as and when required, and that any organisation and work practices issues are identified and addressed.

The main considerations governing whether or not a decision is made to outsource such services as information systems and services include:

- Need to concentrate on the core business of the organisation without distraction by infrastructure issues
- Strategic importance of information — elements that are perceived more strategically important to the business are generally less likely to be outsourced
- Efficiency and effectiveness of current services in this domain — there may be considerable benefit in outsourcing an operation that is not well run in-house
- Where the environment is less stable and there may be rapid changes, it is generally not considered desirable to outsource the services

Advantages of outsourcing may include:

- Cost reduction, especially if the in-house operation was inefficient
- Staffing flexibility, enabling the organisation to gain the benefit of a range of specialised skills and personnel, and to have access to more or less staff as may be required, but without having to employ them full time
- Focus on the services required, rather than the logistics of providing them

Outsourcing involves the vesting of considerable trust in the organisation providing the services. In effect it constitutes the creation of a business partnership and would normally be expected to run over a prolonged period. It is quite possible for an outsourced service to present a barrier to development and progress if an effective working relationship has not been established. It is vital that the organisation retains control over direction and development, although it would normally do this in close liaison with its outsourcing partner.

POISE

The procurement of any major computer system is a complex task. In July 1993 the NHS Executive issued new guidelines, known as POISE, which are intended to introduce a standard process for IT procurement across the NHS. POISE stands for Procurement of Information Systems Effectively. The intention has been to provide a flexible process which can be adapted to suit the complexity and characteristics of each procurement.

The aim of POISE is to produce a performance-based contract, rather than a descriptive contract. The difference can be illustrated by an example of producing a specification for exterior painting of woodwork.

> **Performance Specification:** "The woodwork must be protected against all weather and prevented from deterioration; its appearance must be smooth, glossy and brilliant white; it must be guaranteed to retain its appearance for a minimum of five years".
>
> **Descriptive Specification:** "All bare wood or deteriorated existing paintwork must be rubbed down; bare areas must be primed with a non-lead primer; all surfaces must receive two applications of undercoat and one of brilliant white oil-based gloss paint; all work must be evenly applied free from drips and runs".

The descriptive specification looks safer and compels the supplier to do the job in one way only and no other. However, it does not give any guarantee of how long the painting will last. Nor does it allow the supplier to use his technical knowledge to propose a more modern sort of paint that covers in one coat, which could save on labour and lower the cost of the job. Similar arguments can be applied to the supply of information systems.

There are four distinct stages in the POISE procedure: planning, preparation of documents, purchase and performing the contract.

Stage 1. plan procurement

Before procurement is started, ensure that you understand the business justification, expected benefits, resources needed, budget required and that full management approval has been obtained.

1.1 Understand and check the procurement decision (has an investment appraisal been done?)
1.2 Understand the market and availability of solutions (suppliers, prices etc.)
1.3 Agree on a procurement approach and clarify the level of effort that will be required
1.4 Prepare and authorise a procurement plan including:
   • Scope, goals and user requirements
   • Approved budget, authorisation and time-scales
   • Resources (people and facilities) to be made available for procurement process
1.5 Set up a project board, project director and project team with clear accountability and authority.

Stage 2. prepare documents

Documents, such as the statement of need, should articulate business needs, not solutions, and allow the supplier maximum flexibility in proposing his solution. Public procurement rules and good practice must be followed at all times to ensure fair and consistent evaluation of proposals.

2.1 Detailed Statement of Need (DSON) sets out what the project is trying to achieve. DSON forms the basis of subsequent procurement documents. Typical contents include:
  - Introduction and background
  - Business requirements
  - Requirements of the system (this should not be a "wish list")
  - Workload (to allow supplier to size the system)
  - System characteristics (e.g. response time, security etc.)
  - Constraints (e.g. need to interface with existing applications)
  - Evaluation criteria
  - Instructions to suppliers

2.2 Summary of Need (SON) emphasises mandatory needs and key differentiators. This will be the same as DSON for simple projects

2.3 EC advertisement requesting evidence of supplier credibility. All procurements for more than 200,000 ecu (about £160,000) must be advertised in the Official Journal of the European Communities using restricted procurement procedure

2.4 Draft contract framework with outline Statement of Requirements (SOR). The final contract is a summary of agreements reached during procurement and a rule-book for implementation

Stage 3. purchase

3.1 Issue EC advertisement and select credible and capable suppliers based on response to published criteria such as financial stability and technical capability to meet the requirement

3.2 Issue SON and receive proposals from suppliers

3.3 Evaluate suppliers' proposals based on solutions to specified needs. Typical criteria may be:

High level criteria

Lower Level Criteria

Application software

Fit with functional requirements

Proven state of development

Features

Supplier credibility

> Quality/realism of proposal
>
> Attitude during procurement
>
> Financial stability
>
> Track record in similar situations
>
> Reference sites

Project organisation

> Quality of implementation plans
>
> Quality of staff proposed
>
> Ability to meet timetable
>
> QA and change control procedures

System operation/support System support arrangements

> Ease of operation of hardware
>
> System resilience
>
> Facility management/outsourcing (if needed)

Hardware/infrastructure

> Attributes (e.g. backup facilities)
>
> Performance
>
> Compliance with standards
>
> Growth potential
>
> Maintenance/support contract terms

3.4 Produce short-list of preferred suppliers, ensuring that all can meet the need

3.5 Issue Statement of Requirements (SOR), negotiate draft contract and complete detailed schedules, such as:

A. Statement of requirements
B. Contractor's solution
C. Contractor's other responsibilities
D. Authority's responsibilities
E. Timetable
F. Acceptance and completion
G. Financial control
H. Change control
I. Escrow Agreement

Clarify deliverables, roles, responsibilities, time scales and ensure a performance-based contract for tendering

3.6 Tender as per standing orders

3.7 Award to chosen supplier based on most economically advantageous solution over lifetime of project. Notify and debrief unsuccessful suppliers

Stage 4. perform contract

The contract is designed to be a working document that guides implementation.

4.1 Implement contract — supplier and authority each meet their contractual obligations. A sound implementation plan and strong project management can both contribute to a successful implementation

4.2 Monitor and review — any issues, e.g. relating to system acceptance, are identified and managed. Any modifications or extensions to the contract are covered by change control procedures in the contract

4.3 Complete the benefits realisation programme. Measure benefits and feedback into the planning process

Criteria for approving large IT projects

Criteria for approving IT projects costing more than £1 million include demonstrating that:

(1) The investment is an integral part of the local IM&T strategy, based on the local business plan

(2) Benefits (cash-releasing and non-cash-releasing) have been identified and assessed, with commitments from all affected parties to realise them

(3) A formal business case has been set out, based on investment appraisal, showing costs, costable and non-costable benefits; future costs and cash benefits should be discounted to give "net present value"

(4) Option appraisal has been conducted, including assessment of "doing nothing" and of achieving the same benefits from better use of existing investment

(5) There is a clear understanding of the procurement process (based on POISE)

(6) The project will be managed in a structured manner (PRINCE being the NHS standard) with staged review points

(7) Commitments from the chief executive and PRINCE project board chairman indicating each person's role in the procurement, implementation and benefits realisation process

(8) A plan for benefits realisation has been prepared, including assignment of responsibility for realising benefits to a specified person with sufficient authority and resources to deliver

(9) A resourced and structured training programme

(10) Sufficient and adequately skilled IM&T staff are available to manage the specification, procurement and implementation of the system

(11) A commitment given to post-implementation evaluation, results of which shall be made available to the authority approving the investment

Chapter 6   Healthcare administration systems

Patient master index

The Patient Master Index (PMI) provides the administrative foundation for all patient-oriented systems within the hospital. The PMI is an index of all patients who have medical records held at the hospital. It provides the only positive way of matching a patient by name with his or her case-notes, films and reports stored by hospital number.

Prior to introduction of computers, the traditional PMI was maintained as a card index sorted in alphabetical order of patient name, containing the patient's name, address, hospital number, GP and other details. The only way that staff could check patient demographic details and to find case notes (filed by hospital number) was to visit the index or telephone index staff.

On-line VDU access to the patient master index greatly reduces walking and almost eliminates the need for telephone calls. Measured time savings at one hospital resulting from using a multi-user computerised master index available in 15 locations (near but not at most users' place of work) were:

	hrs/week saved
Travel to and from index	19
Time at index	46
Time telephoning index	29
Total time saved/week	94 (approx 2.5 FTE)

Significantly greater time savings are achievable where each medical secretary, ward clerk and clinic receptionist has immediate access to the master index using a VDU at their place of work.

The same study showed a further saving of 2 staff involved in maintaining a manual index, adding new entries, checking for duplicate registrations, maintaining cards in the correct order, answering telephone calls and assisting users.

The quality of computer information is better than on a card index, because computer systems demand complete and consistent data, which can be validated at source. On a card index, important information is often missing, other handwritten information may be illegible, entries may be made in the wrong places and often notes are scribbled in margins or even on the back of the card. For example, in one study on a well run index, 17 per cent of records had important omissions. Manual index cards may need to be removed from the file for updating and can easily be put back in the wrong place. (The rules for placing all of the John Smith's in a consistent order on a large index are quite complex). Misfiling leads to duplicate registrations with two or more sets of notes for these patients, each independent and unknown to the other. In addition, the ability to maintain multiple linkages, for example between family members, is very limited.

An accurate and easily accessible master index minimises delays in finding patient's notes (e.g. in an accident and emergency department). It can contribute towards speeding up the start of a patient's treatment whilst avoiding the hazard of raising a duplicate set of notes. One useful output from the master index is automatic production of patient identification labels for use on forms, specimen bottles and so on.

Issues in PMI design and use

Identification of individuals is one of the key issues underpinning the effective administration of patient care services. This is a significant problem in any information system, manual or computerised.

Where a patient has multiple records, continuity and integrity of care are compromised: information that is known in one record, for example an adverse drug reaction, is unknown to users of the other record(s) for that individual. A fatal error can easily be made.

In many hospitals separate departments may maintain totally separate records (the authors are aware of one institution where up to seven separate records for a single individual could exist, without any pointers or linkages to each other). However, even where there is a single patient master index (PMI), failure to locate the individual on a PMI search inevitably results in a duplicate registration being made. User training is therefore vital.

Confusion over identities may easily arise across PMI boundaries. If every institution assigns different unique identifiers to each individual, there is no easy way of confirming identities of individuals as they pass between providers. More and more data is being sent electronically across these boundaries: it is vital that this should not lead to confusion over identities either when care is provided or when data is being analysed. This is one of the strong arguments for implementation of national and international unique health identifiers.

The converse problem, where the same record is shared by two different individuals, is less common but still of concern. Few individuals would be happy if, for example, they were uncertain as to whether the prescription they had just been given, or the operation that was to be performed, related to their own problem or that of some other person sharing the same name or record number.

There are not infrequent reports in the press of situations where an individual has been subjected to an invasive procedure as a consequence of mistaken identity. This may arise because of the latter problem (single record for multiple individuals), but more often arises because of problems with matching individuals to their records in the process of searching the PMI. It may be compounded when a care provider fails to make the necessary checks to determine that the record he/she has been given belongs to that individual.

It is routine to fix identifiers to inpatients, for example round one wrist or ankle, to ensure that they can be readily identified, especially when totally dependent (e.g. unconscious, unable to speak). Some institutions have recently taken to fixing two such tags to each individual to avoid the confusion that arises if one is lost — there are still too many incidents where this happens and, for example, babies are given to the wrong parents. Providing computer readable identity tags (e.g. *see* Movement and access control page 84) for patients can provide the necessary infrastructure for tracking them better, linking them with their records and samples, and providing the audit trail to link patient, carer, location and procedure (see security issues — chapter 11).

What identifies an individual?

It is clear that that are numerous characteristics which make an individual unique and distinct from others. We have no difficulty recognising people that we know at a glance. However, to someone who has no knowledge of the individuals concerned, what are the features that can be used to distinguish between them? This is an important issue because it determines what should be stored in the PMI system, how a PMI search should be implemented and what should be displayed to a searcher of the PMI to be checked with the patient.

Names

Most individuals are identified by their names, and names are often seen as the key identifier. It is conventional to separate family name from given name(s). In most European societies the given names precede the family name — for example "John Frederick Smith" where *Smith* is the family name and *John* and *Frederick* are given names. However, structuring a PMI system on the basis of "family name" and "given name(s)" is no longer adequate in the face of increasingly polyglot and multi-cultural societies.

For example, those of Asian origin commonly adopt the reverse convention, where the family name is the first to be presented in their naming convention — for example "Pang Heng Chung" where *Pang* is the family name and *Heng* and *Chung* are given names. Some may add a "European" style name at the end, for example "Pang Heng Chung James".

Many societies use prefixes to names, for example "de Boer" or "van der Woude" or "von an der Lan". In Arab societies the prefixes Al- and El- (with or without hyphens) may be used before virtually any family name, and the short words "bin" or "abu" inserted at various points. These raise the issue as to how many given names are required to identify an individual, and how to deal with the prefixes and other names.

Names may be spelled in different ways, and pronounced in ways that are not immediately linked to their spelling (for example, *Johnathan* or *Jonathon*, *Smith* or *Smythe* and *Cholmondley* (which may be pronounced "Chumly") or *Cockburn* (pronounced "Coburn") or *St.John* (pronounced "Sinjun")). Names that are normally written in other character sets (e.g. Chinese, Japanese, Arabic, Indian) may not be directly spellable in our alphabet, and there are often several equally appropriate ways of representing them (the converse is of course true when we travel to countries using different alphabets).

There is the issue of name stability. Many individuals change their names by choice, by contract (e.g. marriage) or by formal declaration. They also commonly change the name by which they prefer to be known, which is not necessarily the first of their given names. In some societies individuals change their names, taking on that of an ancestor when that ancestor dies.

Finally there is the problem of keystroke errors. Approximately one keystroke in 20 is erroneous, based on large scale surveys. A full name is likely, therefore, to have approximately 2 keying errors as entered and without any form of checking. A simple search of the PMI database may fail to find the individual if the "string" entered is significantly different from that which is stored.

Address

Addresses are usually stored in PMI systems for three reasons. First in order to send correspondence and accounts to the individual, second as a means of identifying the individual, and third for research and grouping according to domicile.

There are substantial variations in address structures. For example compare the addresses below:

P.O.Box 593	Flat 15	Appartement 109
Cheltenham	Beaulieu Mansions	Batiment C
Glos.	Amiens Way	110–119 Rue de la Misericorde
	South Street	F-1019 Chartres-11
	Near Boughton	France
	Sunderland SU1 8NZ	

It is not immediately easy to "parse" these into equivalent sub-units. This may mean that address is represented in a relatively unstructured way and as such is not suitable for searching. On the other hand rules and structures can be set down which permit standard formats to be identified, so facilitating searching and sorting.

One approach is that of "tagging" address elements with a code that identifies what sort of an element it is. For example *Beaulieu Mansions* or *Batiment C* would be tagged as "buildings", whilst *Cheltenham, South Street* and *Chartres-11* would be tagged as towns. This could make the process of executing a search more complicated since any address element may be placed in any database field, and the element and tag may have to be searched together. Once again the problem of keying errors complicates the issue.

Addresses are less stable than names. About 10 per cent of the population moves address in any one year, and some individuals move much more frequently. An address entry that was recorded 5 or more years ago may not even be recognised by the individual themselves.

Some level of address verification may be useful as a means of partial validation of entries. For example, a prompt may be set up to seek a town name, province/county name and postcode: these can each be checked against lists, and checked for internal consistency before the entries are accepted. This may be useful in improving data quality, especially on a national PMI system, and may be able to contribute markedly to the ease of searching (e.g. for a postcode or town name) and sorting for analysis.

Date of birth

Date of birth can be a valuable field for identification. Dates of birth do not change. Some people do not know their own date of birth, or are unwilling to reveal it, and many do not know the exact birthdate of a friend or relative whom they may be accompanying to a hospital. Nevertheless, dates of birth are relatively reliable.

However, there are several different ways of representing dates in widespread use, with the components in different orders, some in words, others in numerals, using various abbreviations (e.g. Dec), languages (e.g. Juillet) and delimiters between elements (e.g. / . , : – etc.). The format adopted by the International Standards Organisation (ISO) is ccyymmdd, i.e. 19460522 for the 22nd of May 1946.

Sex

Even sex is not as stable an element as one might suppose. For a start there are not just 2 sexes — most systems permit at least 3 (male, female, unknown), and some add a fourth (indeterminate

— meaning that gender cannot definitively be assigned). The ISO standard has four categories:

0 – unknown
1 – male
2 – female
9 – unspecified

Where older databases are being upgraded, or merged, the number of "unknowns" may be quite large either because the source system did not record sex, or because the data is unreliable. Database searches should always include the "unknowns" and "unspecifieds" in all searches in order to minimise the chance of missed matches. Assigning sex on the basis of names is unwise, since many names may be used by either sex.

Of course individuals do also change sex, but not very frequently.

Identity number

The use of a unique identifier is the only sure way to ensure that no confusion arises. All that is then required is for the various attributes of that individual (names, aliases, address, sex etc.) to be kept up to date at each care encounter, and the updates to be notified to a central server so that other systems are able to update their local indexes as required. The unique identifier for an individual should remain unchanged from birth until death, and numbers should not be reused after the death of an individual.

The need for a unique identifier for an individual, patient or provider, is highlighted in situations where data is stored in multiple distributed data stores, each of which has adopted its own approach to identification, and has applied its own reference number to that individual. The growing practice of exchanging data electronically requires that there is a common identification mechanism, such as a unique identifier. Identifiers will, in the near future, need to be prefixed with a country code as care networks extend internationally. The NHS is moving imminently to introduce a new identity number for all UK residents.

In itself a unique identifier introduces no real threat to privacy. The existence of an individual is seldom a secret. However there are some risks which may be associated with the use of a unique identifier.

- Access to any personal data held in association with the identifier must be restricted to those with a need to know, and with appropriate authorisation: all the data is personal and private and must be respected as such
- Personal privacy may be placed at risk if the health unique identifier is used also for other purposes (e.g. by social security, inland revenue or community services), and/or where data matching is carried out without proper oversight or verification

- Concern arises where provision of care services is made contingent upon presentation of an identification number or token, which may be in conflict with basic human rights
- If the identifier is intrinsically meaningful, private and confidential, information may be inferred simply from scrutiny of the identifier.

These issues, and others, are explored further in Chapter 11 on personal privacy protection.

Searches

Given the foregoing, it is clear that finding a record for an individual is not easy unless a unique identifier has been used and is known to the individual. Most searching systems make use of one or more of the following techniques for improving the "hit rate".

- "Soundex" matching, which searches for strings that sound similar to that which has been entered as the basis for a search
- Partial matches, which assume that the string entered is the leading segment of what may be a much longer name or address
- Range specification, which allow the searcher to enter an approximate date of birth, and/or specify an age range (e.g. aged 20–40 years)
- Algorithms at the database level which ensure, for example, that all name fields are searched for a match, so that, for example, entry of the string "John Smith" will return John J. Smith, Albert John Smith, Charles Frances John Smith as matches, and any alias registrations that include these names, together with all soundex matched variants
- Data verification so as to ensure that elements of the address are validated against tables, e.g. for town, county, postcode etc.
- Permitting the user to initiate a search based on any combination of elements that appear more stable and likely to return the minimum number of hits
- Verification with the individual concerned that the details displayed do indeed relate to themselves, updating where appropriate

For making new registrations on the PMI, other general rules include:

- Refusing permission for a new registration where details are identical to another existing registration
- Requiring a recheck where variations from an existing registration (or alias) are minimal

There is a pressing need for the worldwide use of unique identifiers for patients, providers and care institutions/facilities. Increasing mobility of individuals and development of care teams means that there is a rapidly increasing chance that a care encounter will involve a provider-patient pair who have never met one another before. The risks of errors arising out of mistaken identity are already very significant.

Electronic communications between care sector bodies require that the identities of patient, provider and institutions be unambiguously specified. Without this it would, for example, be asking too much of a provider to accept the opinions of another provider whose identity he/she was unable to establish, or to expect a payer to fund care for an individual whose identity they were unable to confirm.

Searching for any of these entities without a unique identifier is tedious, especially where the database is large (for example a national PMI, which would have millions of entries and would return thousands of "hits" for common names such as John Smith).

Hospital Information Support Systems (HISS)

The development of HISS (Hospital Information Support Systems) is based on the demonstrated need for an information communications and management system that supports the needs of care providers and administrators within the hospital. HISS is:

an IT environment which meets the real-time (immediate processing) operational and information needs of health professionals who deliver care to patients, whilst also providing accurate and timely information for management purposes.

Note the use of the word *environment*. HISS provides an infrastructure that allows separate applications to communicate and share information by working together. Implementation of a HISS is not just about installing networks and computers, but is concerned with changing information flows throughout the hospital. This has implications for almost everyone working there.

Implementations of HISS may be considered at three levels:

1. Patient Master Index (PMI): a population based register including a unique identifier and maintaining records of demographic data, such as patient name, address, date of birth and GP details across all applications.
2. Results inquiry: a system providing access to each patient's administrative and clinical information (such as test results) at terminals throughout the institution, on wards and in laboratories and clinics.
3. Order communications system (OCS): an electronic requesting and order entry system. Clinical and other (e.g. catering, linen) orders may be made from terminals on wards and in clinics, with automatic forwarding of requests to relevant departments and systems. Results and reports are made available on wards and in clinics as soon as they are prepared by the laboratory.

Hospitals can implement a HISS using either a step-by-step (incremental) or a "big-bang" approach. The incremental approach builds on existing investments, but may face problems in developing interfaces between old and incompatible systems. The crux of the problem is that two systems can only ever exchange data that is genuinely common to both. This problem is serious, but it should soon be alleviated by use of standards for healthcare data interchange. The big bang approach involves major expenditure all at once and a massive management of change problem. Frequently all the business may be placed with a single supplier, who may or may not subscribe to a modular environment, open systems and standards. If the system installed is neither modular nor standards compliant, the purchaser will probably be locked in to that systems supplier for any future development, extension or modification, which may prove both limiting and expensive.

Patient administration systems

The central computer application in most hospitals is a Patient Administration System (PAS) or patient management system (PMS). This provides the link between the patient identity and their medical record number, admissions to hospital, the medical officers responsible for care, attendance at clinics and so on. The PAS maintains the patient master index, tracks inpatients, manages the admission waiting list, and contributes to service contract management.

The impact of PAS has usually been restricted to the central medical records department. Other hospital staff have complained that investment in PAS has provided them with few direct benefits in their day-to-day work. Such criticisms often reflect a lack of understanding of what PAS sets out to achieve and of the scale of organisational changes that are required if all of the potential benefits are to be realised.

The central medical records department originally became the nerve centre for hospital information because of the need for a single source of patient information. The only way that this can be done with manual systems is to centralise the information required for each function, so that all relevant records and files are maintained in one location.

The multi-user capability of a PAS computer removes the logical requirement for centralised physical records. PAS permits updating and display of information from any terminal or workstation connected to it. Decentralisation of patient administration functions to wards, clinics and medical secretaries, away from the central medical records department, presents management with challenge of organisation development and training which have yet to be widely grasped.

The scale of potential productivity benefits obtainable from PAS has been estimated in evaluation studies. The following figures for saving full time equivalent staff (FTE) are based on work study data in a 750 bed hospital.

Application	Saving (FTE)
Patient master index maintenance	2
Use of master index (indirect savings)	2.5
Bed state maintenance	1
Inpatient coding and statistics	3
Waiting list maintenance	1
Waiting list statistics	2
Outpatient appointments	3.5
	15.0

Inpatients

Inpatient modules maintain details of the hospital's bed state and location of patients in hospital, as well as providing statistical returns. Bed state is derived from ward returns which show all patients who have been admitted, transferred, discharged or died (ADT) since the previous return. Once in the computer, this information can be sorted to display patients in alphabetic order, by bed order within ward, or to identify empty beds.

The patient location facility provides a service for friends and relatives, GPs and outside organisations. The capacity to find an individual quickly by patient name or hospital number helps all who need to know the whereabouts of patients, including the telephone switchboard, front reception, post room, porters and patients' property office. Printed ward lists in bed order are used by ward clerks, nurses and kitchen staff. Lists of patients and their locations are used by doctors to find all those for whom they are responsible, especially those in outlying wards or temporary locations.

On-line bed state data shows empty beds to help admissions office and on-take doctors identify available beds. Hospital managers can monitor admissions policy and waiting lists on a day-to-day basis, and can maintain bed occupancy at a level at which the hospital functions most efficiently.

Computer-based bed status systems have taken the place of traditional wall-mounted ward bed boards which showed occupancy of every bed in the hospital, together with an alphabetic cross-reference card index, which showed the location of each in-patient. Such manual systems were error prone and time consuming.

The inpatient system also provides hospital statistics which saves a substantial amount of clerical time. The clerical effort involved in coding and keying administration details required by central returns for every in-patient episode by hand is considerable. There are also major concerns over quality of data captured by retrospective coding.

The problems of clinical coding are discussed later under "Coding and Classification" (Chapter 9).

Waiting lists

Computer-based waiting list systems provide benefits to patient and clinicians. Anxiety for patients and their relatives is reduced if the patient is kept well informed about the likely admission date. Instant access to the waiting list on a VDU screen helps medical secretaries and other staff answer queries quickly from GPs and patients. Streamlining procedures to issue TCI (to come in) letters saves secretarial time and gives the patient extra notice.

Decentralised computerised waiting lists save clinicians time in visiting the central admissions office and make it easier to take account of nursing load and operation list constraints. The computer displays the waiting-list for each specialty by priority and length of time on the waiting list. Details of each patient's proposed operation and any special factors can be checked. When patients are selected to come in, the computer prints all of the lists, letters, and admission forms. Internal enquiries are reduced because wards and front reception are provided with lists in advance, giving them all relevant details of each expected admission.

If a patient refuses an offer of admission for some reason, the computerised waiting list makes it easy to select the most appropriate short-notice patient and to produce all of the necessary documentation with the minimum of effort. Similarly, if the hospital needs to cancel an admission, work required is simplified. Errors are reduced because data is entered once only, and subsequent transcription errors are avoided. A major benefit of any computerised waiting list system is automatic production of detailed monthly statistics subdivided by specialty, area of residence and type of purchaser in the form required by the Department of Health. In some hospitals more than 300 separate returns need to be prepared each month.

Outpatient appointments

An essential requirement of any appointments system is that there should be only one record for each appointment. In a manual system this is normally recorded in a diary for each separate clinic, facility or doctor. Such an appointments diary can only be used by one person at a time, and has to be kept in only one physical location. This leads to specialisation amongst appointment clerks, and queues of patients waiting to make appointments with one clerk while others may be underemployed.

An on-line computerised appointments system allows any authorised person to make an appointment. Each member of staff has access to the master diary held in the computer. For example, when a patient is discharged, ward staff can book the first follow-up appointment then and there, and confirm it with the patient. It is quick and easy to check the date and time of any patient's next appointment.

Clinic appointment lists are printed sorted by name, by hospital number or by time of appointment, and used for checking patients in, picking case-notes and arranging ambulance transport. The computerised appointments system monitors each patient's flow through the system, recording time of appointment, time that the patient arrived, time seen and time of departure. This allows standards of service to be measured against those set out in the Patient's Charter. The doctor can use a VDU in the consulting room to see the list of patients waiting to be seen, and can select the next patient by pressing a single key.

After each clinic, letters may be sent out automatically to confirm appointments and to offer fresh appointments to those who did not attend (DNA). Regular statistics are produced automatically.

This leads to decentralisation of out-patient appointments and re-deployment of staff currently employed in centralised appointments offices. The need to produce additional statistical returns in future, to meet the needs of contracting and of the Patient's Charter is likely to increase the volume of statistical analysis of out-patient appointments.

Assets register

Most institutions have large investment in equipment and other assets. These assets will be distributed in various locations, and may be moved from place to place as required. Equipment may be acquired through a large variety of mechanisms, including grants, trust funds and donations. But the cost and burden of support and maintenance (typically amounting to between 10 and 15 per cent of purchase price per annum), and of replacement (adding a further 20–25 per cent of the purchase price per annum) almost always falls on the institution however the assets were originally acquired.

Tracking these resources is vital in order to minimise the number required and thus the overall cost. All must be maintained in working order, upgraded as necessary and replaced when they reach the end of their economical working life. An assets register and tracking system is a key part of the management infrastructure of any modern healthcare organisation, and can contribute significantly to minimising unnecessary expenditure.

Rostering

Rostering systems ensure that an appropriate quantity of staff are scheduled for each activity, and that their skills mix is appropriate to the tasks to be undertaken. It is wasteful to assign too many staff, or staff with more skills than are required: it is dangerous to assign inadequate numbers of staff, or those whose skills and competencies are insufficient for the requisite tasks.

These issues become particularly important in the management of operating theatres, special procedures facilities and in assigning nursing staff to the wards. A secondary advantage is that the systems can be used in making decisions about staff promotions and rewards, since all attendances, activities and responsibilities are recorded.

Movement and access control

Tracking the movements of materials, such as notes and X-rays, has proven notoriously time consuming. Some PAS systems provide a facility for noting where objects are, but their manual nature means they are often poorly maintained. The use of bar codes is invaluable, and can readily be set up on a single PC for the entire institution. Every object to be tracked is assigned a code, together with every receiving location or person. Multiple copies of the bar code are printed on sticky labels on the object, and each time it is moved, one copy is peeled off and attached to a daily return sheet, together with a bar code for the sender and receiver. The returns are scanned centrally, and in this way the objects can readily be tracked.

Most institutions have implemented identity card systems, normally including a name and photograph, and often also a bar code, magnetic strip or smart chip. These can be used to afford access to restricted areas, as well as to identify an individual. Creating an integrated security system whereby the same token is used for access to the computer system also (see Chapter 11) has many advantages.

Resource monitoring

Effective and efficient administration is essential to the success of any healthcare unit: however good the care it may provide, it can only prosper by being competitive and efficient in managing its business. Efficient use of all the resources at its disposal is essential.

Central to this is the capacity to track objects and people, and to schedule timings. Effective tracking and scheduling can have a big impact on efficiency and performance. Considerable time is wasted in trying to find objects, for example notes or images, that have gone astray, and in locating staff, equipment and patients. Resources can only be used efficiently where there is an effective appointments system in place to ensure full use of staff and plant, and where rostering ensures that an adequate number of staff with the appropriate mix of skills are available to carry out the necessary work (e.g. in theatre, on the ward, in the clinic).

Tracking

Objects and people need to be tracked in order to maximise their availability, facilitate their movements and minimise the risk of loss (e.g. of notes or films). It is important to record encounters and interactions between, for example, patients with providers, or patients and equipment in order to track the provision of services, identify costs, prepare billing information and review staff workloads and facility utilisation.

Examples of such tracking requirements include:

- Tracking patients and staff as they move about the facility to enable communication and to record encounters
- Tracking such items as patient samples, records and radiographs and their association with individuals and locations to ensure that accessibility is maximised, losses are minimised, and individuals are accountable
- Tracking relationships and encounters between patients and medical officers or nurses
- Registering moveable assets (e.g. laptop computers, overhead projectors etc.) and keeping track of them
- Stock control, and tracking inwards and outwards movements of materials in stores and all other areas (e.g. sterile theatre packs, ward supplies and drugs etc.)
- Tracking resource utilisation by specific patients, to assign costs to the unit responsible for their care, or billing the patient/payer direct
- Providing activity status/reports for items of major equipment, and bed occupancy; calculating costs per service provided and identifying less profitable resources/assets/lines of business

Security and audit trails

Some areas of an institution house equipment that is especially valuable or easily removed (e.g. computers), or contain information that is particularly sensitive (e.g. medical records) or present a risk unless special precautions are observed (e.g. radioactivity, infection, barrier units).

Entry to and departure from these areas may need to be monitored or restricted to authorised individuals. Sensing devices can be used to permit entry: where the risks are especially high, a keypad can be provided for entry of a password as a means of authenticating the holder of a token. Alternatively equipment may be tagged and sensors installed to detect its movement through gates.

Administration of medication and performance of procedures, especially invasive or risky procedures on patients, must be ordered and carried out only by authorised staff. These activities must all be logged since they may subsequently become the focus of litigation.

Scheduling activities and usage

Expensive equipment and facilities, such as scanners and operating theatres, should be used at near full capacity in order to achieve maximum business efficiency. Staff should be rostered and encounters with patients be planned by appointment or booking systems for optimal productivity.

Assisting maintenance

Service histories must be kept for all equipment, especially equipment where a malfunction may cause loss of life, such as X-ray equipment, ventilators, infusion pumps, intensive care monitors etc. Every fault must be logged, and an audit trail of repair sign-offs by supervisors obtained. Costs need to be allocated to the "owner" of the equipment.

The running costs and anticipated useful life for major items of plant and equipment need to be known and factored in to budgets to ensure that sufficient funds are allocated in advance for this purpose.

Unique identification

In some institutions almost everything that moves and most things that do not are assigned identifiers, usually based on bar codes. Movements and associations between individuals and facilities or services can readily be recorded using bar code scanners, together with time stamps in order to obtain a comprehensive view of activities and resource utilisation.

An alternative approach involves the use of tokens, such as magnetic stripe cards that can readily be recognised by a computer. These can be swiped through readers at strategic locations, and can be supplemented with a password for holder authentication where access to sensitive areas and secure facilities is required.

Recently a third approach has been introduced based on the "active badge" concept. Staff are provided with an electronic badge which is activated by infra-red transmitters in strategic locations. The badge replies by emitting its unique code using a radio frequency, rather like the transponder on a civil aircraft when it is interrogated by radar. This enables individuals to be located as they move about. Calls can be diverted to the nearest telephone and messages can be displayed on the nearest computer terminal.

Various entity complexes need to be assigned unique identifiers. One such example is a "clinic": this can be held in any location and conducted by any appropriate provider on any assigned date and time. However the clinic (identified by date, time and place) needs to be assigned a unique identifier so that staff and patients can be scheduled to conduct/attend it.

Chapter 7 Contract and resource management

Health care service providers and agencies are now in direct competition with each other for business. Their survival is increasingly dependent upon being able to attract customers. The ability to attract business in turn depends upon both clinical and business performance.

The central concept of the internal healthcare market is that there is a funder who supplies the money, a purchaser who ultimately authorises payment, and a provider who delivers the service to the customer or patient. The provider is responsible to the purchaser for the quality of the service provided. The chain of purchaser and provider runs right through the system. The full picture is quite complex, but to give one example, the purchaser-provider chain from the taxpayer to the provision of a laboratory test may pass from:

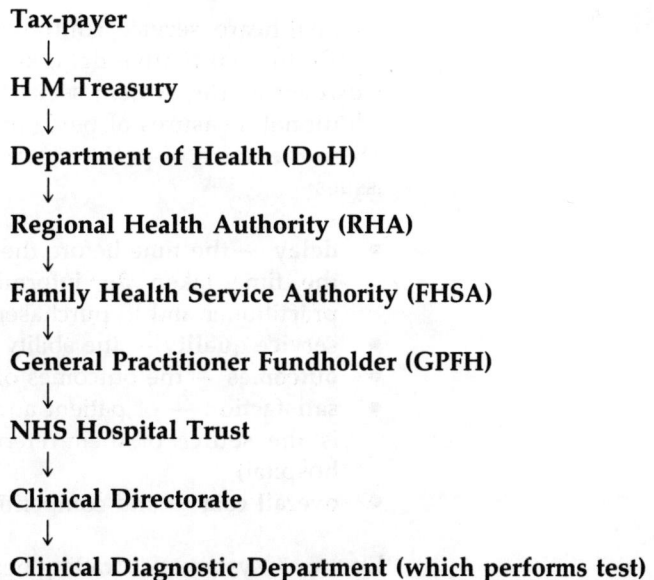

Tax-payer
↓
H M Treasury
↓
Department of Health (DoH)
↓
Regional Health Authority (RHA)
↓
Family Health Service Authority (FHSA)
↓
General Practitioner Fundholder (GPFH)
↓
NHS Hospital Trust
↓
Clinical Directorate
↓
Clinical Diagnostic Department (which performs test)

Figure 7.1

Establishing contracts

Each link in the chain involves a contract which specifies the quantity and quality of service to be provided and price to be paid. If a purchaser is to work this system effectively, he/she needs information from each potential provider to enable the price and quality of service offered to be assessed and compared when making contracts. Some idea of the quantity that will be required over the next year is valuable in negotiation of quantity discounts, and in ensuring that the required provider capacity is there.

Subsequently the purchaser needs to assess value obtained. The service provider must furnish the purchaser with sufficient information to assess the quantity and quality of the services provided. Inevitably those providers who supply purchasers with the information required and are able to back up their claims with auditable performance figures will win business and those that do not will lose out. Purchasers will be more inclined to place their business with units which are able to offer guarantees of availability and value for money.

The survival of provider units depends on the value of contracts they win. Information is power. The need to attract and keep contracts is forcing hospitals to provide purchasers with whatever information they require. For example, fund-holding GPs and District Health Authorities are demanding and getting formal assurances about speed of issue of clinic letters and discharge summaries and more information on in-patient and out-patient waiting times.

Contract performance

As healthcare service contracting grows, attention is paid principally to quantitative data, such as patient throughput statistics. However as the system seeks to achieve better value for money, additional measures of performance and quality will be required. These measures of performance are likely to relate to the following issues:

- **delay** — the time before the required services can be provided; the time taken for information to be supplied to referring practitioner and to purchaser
- **service quality** — the ability to provide high standard services
- **outcomes** — the outcomes of care services provided
- **satisfaction** — of patient and of the referring professional (who is the source of their referrals, and therefore a client of the hospital)
- **overall cost** — and competitiveness

Electronic systems for trading healthcare services will be established. Providers with capacity available will offer these to purchasers through longer term contracts for the future supply of services, or through immediate and short term availability in a "spot market". The spot market prices will reflect the laws of supply and demand and may be lesser or greater than contract prices. They will provide the customer with a choice of when and where elective services are provided. They will also offer the referring doctor the convenience of being able at once to locate where an acute bed is available for emergency care. As all sectors of the healthcare environment become more cost-conscious, these trading systems will provide an essential service to purchasers, providers and consumers alike.

Information systems are required to support these clinical and business requirements. Information is essential to assist in achieving improvements in efficiency and effectiveness in both clinical and business performance, and in recording these data in a form that is amenable to verification and audit.

Case-mix

Defining "products" of healthcare services

A key issue facing each provider is to specify precisely what it is that they are selling. The product of any hospital or clinic is individual patient care, involving provision of a selection of services designed to diagnose, assess and/or treat the patient. However, no two patients are ever exactly the same and so a method is needed to classify broadly similar patients into groups, and to provide a profile of the mix of cases managed by a service unit ("case-mix").

The basis for classifying the patients into groups is determined by the purposes for which this information is being collected. The primary need for the information relates to financial administration and fulfilment of contracts: thus the primary basis for definition of the groups relates to the overall costs and resources consumed in caring for that class of patient.

Case-mix groups

Various systems have been devised for case-mix classification. In general terms each grouping system identifies expected care profiles for each group based on large scale statistical analyses, and indicates a weighting based on the expected level/complexity of care and services required, and a figure for the average length of stay (LOS) expected for the "typical" acute case. Studies are conducted to analyse current costs and care patterns for patients in each category from selected healthcare institutions, and these data are used to revise casemix groupers every year. These revisions take into account changes in technology and improvements in care practices that are continually being made.

Resource groupings and systems are discussed in greater detail under classification and coding systems (chapter 9).

Case-mix and unit funding

The NHS Resource Management Initiative, launched in 1987, set out to introduce contemporary management accountancy techniques into the health service, including budgetary control, standard costing and analysis of variance.

For many years, hospital management was based on block funding of each provider unit. Control was imposed simply by capping the overall budget allocation to that unit. The problem with this system was that it did not reward efficiency — in fact it tended to favour the less efficient units. The typical course of an inpatient care event is that costs are high at the start, when most of the tests and procedures are being undertaken. As the patient recovers and convalesces the daily costs of care fall. Thus a unit that manages to reduce length of stay suffers because the average cost of care per patient-day rises: by contrast, a unit that keeps patients longer than is required benefits inappropriately because the cost of care per patient-day is reduced, as is the workload for staff.

The new approach is based on casemix, where the emphasis is on efficiency and effectiveness of care. Case-mix management focuses attention on the costs involved in treating similar types of patient (case-mix budgets). Contracts are based on case-mix and a fixed price is assigned to each case in a specific group: the larger the number of patients successfully treated, the greater the budgetary allocation to that service unit.

The course of the illness and treatment of each and every patient is unique and is determined by the specific diagnosis, complications that arise, response of that individual to the treatment regimen, and to the options and preferences of that patient.

Case-mix management is normally carried out by computer systems which bring together the information required, including details of tests, procedures and treatments that can be costed for each patient. Much of the data required by a case-mix management system should be provided by other operational systems for patient administration (PAS), clinical information (CIS), medical audit, nursing, laboratory, radiology, pharmacy and theatre management. However, transfer of data from these feeder systems to a case-mix management system requires suitable interfaces and validation of data. This is often not a trivial task.

Standard costs can be built up for each case-mix group. Actual care patterns and costs may then be compared with expected care profiles, standard costs and budgets. The focus of attention should be on management by exception, examining where and why there are significant variations from expected profiles and costs of caring for patients in specific groups. This process should lead doctors to examine their working practices, leading ultimately to improved patient care.

Case-mix code allocation is performed by assembling the required information, usually from discharge notes, coding the data using either ICD9 or Read coding systems and computing the relevant group from tables. When new grouper code tables are produced each year, all that is required is that the new tables are loaded into the software to replace the old: the rest of the system remains unchanged.

Resource management considers hospital management in terms of case-mix groups, that is, groups of patients requiring broadly similar treatment and resource requirements when treated in hospital (iso-resource groups). In the NHS these are are called Healthcare Resource Groups (HRGs)[1]: they are similar in concept to American DRGs (Diagnosis Related Groups) which have formed the basis of US hospital funding since the early 1980s.

Clinical perspectives

Case-mix grouping is not generally welcomed by clinicians. There is a feeling amongst them that every case is unique, and that the rich variety of clinical cases cannot be reduced into such groups without loss of fidelity. Whilst statistically the groups may be accurately described and profiled, there is a clinical perception that "my" cases are more complex or the illnesses further advanced or more severe. Clinicians would prefer to be rewarded on the basis of the amount of effort expended on a case, that is on the basis of fee-for-service. However, where such systems of funding are used, it is difficult to prevent routine over-servicing of patients, since in a specific instance almost any pattern of servicing can be justified on the basis of "clinical judgement".

There is evidence from some institutions that case-mix funding may lead to patients being selected for treatment based on an assessment that their profitability is higher and the risks of complications lower than the norm. In the extreme, and unless special provisions are made, those cases that are known to be high risk or particularly complex or severe will be rejected for care on the basis that they must result in losses being sustained by the service organisation as well as adversely affecting their outcome statistics and reducing their chances of renewing favourable contracts. Organisations that accept such cases out of humanitarian concern will find themselves disadvantaged.

There is also some evidence of degrees of misrepresentation, ranging from slight exaggeration to deliberate misassignment of groups, but this will exist in any system of classification that has financial consequences. In some environments software has even been developed to assist in this process of misclassification.

---

[1]HRGs are being developed by the National Case Mix Office, 1 St Cross Road, Winchester SO23 9AJ, tel 0962 844588.

Data collection and quality

It is generally accepted that there is a need for information of this type in order to monitor contracts and build in appropriate incentives for effectiveness and efficiency. The problem is what information, and of what quality. It is vital that the data supplied is of the highest quality. However, studies of data quality in hospital returns have indicated error levels of up to 50 per cent — hardly a basis for quality administration.

The task of the funder and purchaser is to ensure that national health service policy is followed and to disburse the available funds in pursuance of policy. They must also monitor for evidence of fraud or inappropriate practices, since any approach to healthcare funding has loopholes that may be exploited. To do this they require accurate and adequate information, and techniques for auditing the consistency and validating the quality of that data.

An entire data set relating to a single episode of illness may require contributions from several different data collectors (e.g. GP, admissions office, pathology service, discharge note etc., etc.). Each collector of data needs to be able to perform their piece of the task independently, although possibly in a predetermined sequence so that data collected by one can be made use of, and expanded upon where appropriate by those who follow. Each collector should know the purpose of the data, and be in a position to make informed decisions relating to it.

Some key principles for obtaining quality data for the information system are:

- Ensuring strong and clear links between business goals and data gathering
- Recording of data once only, as close to the source as possible, preferably by the individual responsible for its collection
- Use of only that data which is used, valued and validated at the local level, and is derived from operational systems

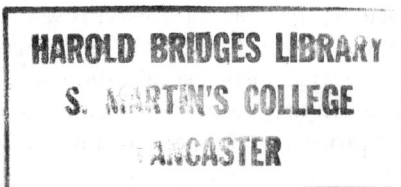

Chapter 8   Clinical systems

Paper records

The conventional approach to keeping patient records in manilla folders is far from ideal. Howard Bleich (1993) has commented:

> *The medical record is an abomination . . . it is a disgrace to the profession that created it. More often than not the chart is thick, tattered, disorganised and illegible; progress notes, consultant's notes, radiology reports and nurses notes are all co-mingled in accession sequence. The charts confuse rather than enlighten; they provide a forbidding challenge to anyone who tries to understand what is happening to the patient.*[1]

Traditional medical records reflect the myriad of different styles, approaches, vocabularies and personalities of their contributors. Records are often incomplete, with pieces lost or missing. They may be misleading, with pieces that have been wrongly inserted from records of others, and material that is out of date. A paper record can only be used by one person at a time, inhibiting parallel care processes.

The structure and format of a paper record is determined by the author at the time it is written. It almost certainly contains redundant data — the same item recorded several times, while other key items are left out. Conventional records are almost useless as a source of data for research due to inconsistency and incompleteness, as well as the prohibitive cost of searching them and abstracting the relevant data items.

Medical records comprise information from many sources, such as referral letters from GPs, past discharge summaries, investigation reports from laboratories and diagnostic imaging departments, medication charts, nursing records, ECG traces as well as history, examination and progress notes written by each doctor who has cared for the patient. Studies in primary care have shown that nearly 70 per cent of the information in notes originates from outside the practice.

[1]Bleich, H L, 1993, *MD Computing* Vol. 10, no 2, p 70.

Paper medical records contribute to lack of clinical incisiveness. The medical record is the key to improving clinical decision-making. At the consultation the only source of written information available to the doctor is that contained in the patient's notes. If an item cannot be found in the patient's notes there is no way that it can serve to benefit future patient care. A paper record can only be used in one place and by one person at a time, which is often not where it is needed. Once the records are to hand there remains the problem of finding what you want, especially in large files.

Electronic medical records

Electronic records can help doctors to assemble, integrate, sort, retrieve and review key facts already known about the patient, as well as to bring together material from remote sources relating to the patient. Computerised patient records (CPRs) can be accessed by several people at the same time, from any terminal on the network. Electronic records can be structured to meet each user's immediate needs, without redundant data recording. Data collection protocols can ensure the completeness, consistency and validity of the data recorded.

Quality of care benefits

Computer-based records help clinicians by:

1. Improving the quality of and access to patient information
2. Integrating information over time and between settings of care
3. Giving decision support to practitioners

Cost of care benefits

Computer-based records reduce costs by:

1. Reducing redundant tests and services due to unavailability of test results
2. Saving administrative costs by generating reports automatically and electronic submission of claims
3. Enhancing productivity by reducing:
   (a) Time needed to find missing records or wait for records already in use
   (b) Redundant data entry
   (c) Time needed to enter or review data in records
4. Reducing risks to the patient (and thus unnecessary costs of care) arising out of:
   (a) Decisions that are delayed due to inability to find/access information

    (b) Repeating invasive tests/procedures (all procedures carry some risk of morbidity or mortality however small those risks may be)

    (c) Minimising the probability of adverse effects or interactions arising from drugs prescribed by practitioners unaware of the full clinical situation

5. Reducing legal exposure arising out of medical records that are inadequate, incomplete or unable to be found when required

The first place in the UK to adopt paper-less consultation records was a GP surgery at Ottery St Mary near Exeter in about 1976. Today, about 600 GPs (2 per cent) no longer keep hand-written notes and the Department of Health has undertaken to change the law to allow computer-based records to be legal as the principal record of care. The use of computerised patient records is likely to increase rapidly during the next few years. By the year 2000 most GPs should be using computerised patient records.

Trustworthy clinical data is of paramount importance for patient care, medical audit and management. Direct data entry at the time of consultation has the advantage that the data is validated by the clinician responsible and can be made immediately available for other clinical and administrative purposes. This, in turn, increases commitment to ensure the accuracy, consistency and completeness of computerised records.

In contrast, whenever data is entered later by clerical or coding staff from handwritten notes made at the time, there is a much greater chance that errors will arise.

CPR content and organisation

A computerised patient record may be large, containing thousands of separate items of information. It is a collection of statements about the patient, and often about relatives and contacts, and may comprise any mix of observations, hearsay, interpretations, actions, orders, reflections, opinions and other miscellaneous entries. There is no limit to the number of such records relating to what has been heard, seen, thought and done by and of the doctors, nurses and others who have attended the patient.

The patient record comprises text, images and audio material, as well as incoming correspondence (which may be scanned into an image format). The electronic record should be multimedia, with image and sound files linked to the text. All the material relating to a single patient has to be linked together and conveniently accessed from the same source.

The large size of computerised patient records presents difficulties for the designer of the user interface. A traditional VDU screen has only 24 lines. One solution is to provide multiple "views" into the patient record, allowing users to display clinical information on the screen in the way that best fits their needs. For example, the Abies Clinical Information System provides the following views:

- The *Summary View* displays the patient's demographic details, lists current problems and clinical episodes and indicates what other information has been recorded by highlighting relevant section headings
- The *Chronological View* of the patient's record allows the doctor to see all the information held in the patient's record presented in reverse chronological order with the most recent data presented first. A variant displays the dates of each encounter
- The *Episode or Problem View* helps the doctor to focus just on entries relating to one individual clinical problem or episode, along the lines of the Problem Oriented Medical Record (POMR) as described by Weed. This is helpful for complex patients with multiple problems and complications, showing the history, tests and treatment for each condition separately
- The *Note Type View* allows doctors to look separately at particular classes of information held in the patient's record. For example the doctor can look at all diagnoses, medication, drug sensitivities or surgical operations
- *Reminders* show overdue procedures follow-up and recall, plus prompts for data missing from the patient record according to predefined protocols

CPR element interrelationships

The structure of any medical record is complex, and its meaning depends on both its structure and its content. It is often important to indicate why a particular procedure was ordered and the context or problem(s) to which it relates (see notes on PROMIS and POMR in chapter 2). In a paper record this may be implicit from its location, but in a computerised record all such associations need to be made explicit. This is achieved using links between the statements which make up the record.

CPR outputs and reports

The worth of any system depends on its value to the user. The computer improves efficiency and productivity by providing information when, where and in the form required. The time taken by medical secretaries to produce discharge summaries and letters can be cut by two-thirds or more.

Furthermore, time and effort can be dramatically reduced on tasks such as the production of management statistics and audit data. The value to the user can be greatly enhanced by providing facilities to generate reports in the format, coding, layout and presentation that is required.

Decision support

Clinical decisions involve diagnosis, therapy and monitoring. The idea of a decision support system is simply to make appropriate information available to the decision-maker in a timely fashion. This requires a mix of situation-specific and patient-specific information appropriate to each decision.

Decision support systems take on many different forms, ranging from simple reminders (e.g. drug interaction warnings) to complex rule-based artificial intelligence (e.g. automated diagnostic routines).

Much effort has been devoted to development of approaches to automated diagnosis, but so far clinicians have shown little interest in adopting such systems. They perform little better than many clinicians and threaten to take much of the job satisfaction out of medical practice. In any case the clinician has to take final legal responsibility for every decision, and so must be fully satisfied with the entire decision-making process including the assessment of the probabilities of each possible outcome.

On the other hand, systems which offer reminders, warnings (e.g. of drug interactions), suggestions, decision critiques and facilitate access to information are generally acceptable to clinicians, and promise to do much more for overall care quality. The growth of knowledge in the biomedical sciences makes it difficult for clinicians to keep up-to-date in best care practices: rapid changes in the cost and local availability of services, and complexity of administrative procedures promise to make decisions support systems increasingly attractive to users.

Three major forces may drive this process. First is growing concern with costs. Paying agencies, especially under managed care arrangements, are starting to place limits on those services for which they will pay in a given clinical context, and the maximum claims that they will accept. Providers are expected to work within these guidelines: stepping outside them will require authorisation or will not be reimbursed. Pressure will be applied to ensure that providers do not over-service their patients. Second is the increasingly litigious nature of society, which means that every decision and action is subject to scrutiny as to whether it was adequate, timely and appropriate in the context, especially where an untoward outcome results. Third is the self-interest of the provider, who has to run a successful business. Systems which can help identify opportunities to maximise income and minimise the effort involved are likely to be warmly welcomed.

These pressures will converge to define a thin band of what constitutes *"contemporary best quality practice"*: there will inevitably be a wide band for individual discretion, but coupled with a progressively decreasing tolerance for individual idiosyncrasies. Examples of this trend can be seen in the protocols that have been developed by Health Maintenance Organisations and other healthcare bodies in the US, which define what they consider as appropriate in a given clinical context, and require permission is sought before any decision involving significant expenditure is taken.

Decision support systems are likely to become widely adopted. Initially, these systems may be simple structured protocols for collecting the data required to help doctors take decisions about referrals to hospital and choices of tests and therapy and to help managers to administer their organisation better. Such systems need to be tightly integrated into clinical information systems.

Data representation

The above discussions about decision support, and the organisation, searching, sorting and reporting of the electronic record are based on an assumption. The patient record must be stored in a way that permits the computer to "understand" it and to manipulate it in an "intelligent" way so that it can carry out these functions and to link the record data to a knowledgebase. The computer can, of course, never demonstrate understanding or intelligence: however, data can be stored in such a way that a computer can manipulate it according to preset rules which gives the semblance of understanding and intelligent action.

When data is stored as free text or as a scanned image (bitmapped), the computer can do little with it other than to store and retrieve it. Data must be stored in a way that permits computerised manipulation, and this means the use of classification and coding systems for both the data recorded in the patient's record and the information in the knowledge base and logic modules that will be used for decision support.

The process of using "preferred terms", selecting from picking lists or finding codes in other ways may, in some instances, slow down the data entry process. This is especially so where a clinician has a well developed set of handwritten abbreviations, hieroglyphics and sketches that enable him/her to record accurate representations of the situation quickly and compactly (even though such representations often convey little to any other user of the record and thus are useless for shared records). However, not all data needs to be stored, classified and coded: only that information that is required for reuse, or for passing through to some other system (e.g. decision support, reporting) need be classified and coded. The remainder may be stored as free text, audio notes and, indeed, as freehand sketches where appropriate.

The elements which are required in classified and coded form at present are the problem, date, time and reason for encounter, the diagnosis(es) and co-morbidities, orders and medications, since these incur costs and are required for contract, audit and resource management issues. In future there will also be a need to code progress and outcome information, and to add signs and symptoms to facilitate linkage to decision support systems.

Laboratory systems

Clinical laboratory computing represents a microcosm of much of healthcare computing, with lessons to be drawn which are applicable elsewhere. Chemical pathology laboratories were pioneers in healthcare computing and are now pioneering the use of standards for data interchange with GPs and clinical information systems in hospitals. One reason why these systems have been at the leading edge of automation is that, like the banks, most of the data they deal with is expressed in numerical form, and is thus relatively easily automated. A second reason is the enormous volume of tests performed, so that a small time saving on every test provides a large overall saving.

The order flow process for clinical laboratory tests has five key steps:

(1) Prepare request
(2) Obtain test sample
(3) Analyse sample
(4) Interpret results
(5) Deliver report

Samples

Sample acquisition is performed in several different ways. In some cases (e.g. urine specimen, microbiology swab) the requester obtains the sample and sends it to the laboratory. Some samples require specialised collection, preservation or storage procedures (e.g. blood gases, frozen sections), which can lead to problems when incorrect methods are used. Samples may need to be routed to different laboratories and different request forms are required for many of the tests as well as for the different provider units: there is more than sufficient scope for delays and errors. In other instances the sample and request paperwork can become separated resulting in the test being aborted.

The requester has no special knowledge, understanding or interest in the logistic issues relating to the provision of these services, only in speed and quality with which the results are supplied.

The impact of electronic ordering systems can be substantial. A sample can be provided with a label that uniquely links it to the source, patient and doctor, and routes it directly to the relevant laboratory. The request form can be automatically selected based on the test being requested, and therefore the correct data set is provided by the requester. The completion of the electronic request automatically notifies the laboratory when and where the samples can be collected, and allows better forward planning of laboratory activities. Processing of the sample can commence immediately it is received, since all relevant details about tests required and patient identification are passed through to the laboratory at the time of ordering.

Pathology laboratory procedure

Each laboratory operates a routine based on the working day, which is made easier by early arrival and accurate, legible identification of specimens and request forms. Computerised requesting ensures completeness, consistency and legibility of the request.

When the request (and sample) arrives, the laboratory receptionist checks for any problems, such as an unsuitable specimen, and then issues a laboratory accession number which is used for all internal laboratory procedures. The accession number is the link between request and subsequent results.

If the laboratory computer has an interface to the PAS/PMI system then only the patient number need be entered to identify each new patient, otherwise it needs the patient's name, sex, age, consultant etc. Once request details are in the computer, the laboratory daybook (a list of today's work) may be printed.

Worksheets are produced for each type of test. Using manual systems, technicians produce their own worksheets. This can lead to errors when information on one specimen has to be entered on several worksheets for separate test procedures. Computer-printed worksheets save time, ensure that no task is left out and keep a record of sequence of specimens in analysers.

The calculation of test results using a computer instead of manual methods saves considerable time, although most analysers now do calculations automatically. Many analysers have digital interfaces for linking directly into laboratory information systems: in most instances an interface will be required to convert the output of the analyser into a form that can be accepted by the information system, although there is a standard specification that is recognised by a number of vendors (ASTM 1039).

Laboratory computerisation

Computerisation within laboratories is extensive. Most laboratories use equipment that is driven by computers. Modern autoanalysis equipment can perform a large number of tests on a sample using the same piece of equipment. The tests required are programmed into the controller system, and appropriate reagents to perform these are fed into long tubes in the appropriate order, separated by bubbles of air. Sample and reagents come together as programmed, and the results are then read using appropriate technology (e.g. colour change, emission counters, ion probes). This process means that there is often no need to wait for a batch of samples to arrive in order to process them together: there is a continuous flow of samples through the system, which can be programmed to perform any specific set of tests for each individual sample.

Computers can produce a major improvement in turnaround times for almost all routine tests. Efficiency is greatly enhanced where orders are accepted electronically, and the electronic requests can automatically select the required autoanalyser functions. Benefits may be achieved in reducing the time required to accept and catalogue the sample, to instruct the equipment as to analysis required, to present the results for interpretation, and to prepare and disseminate the report. This in turn can lead to earlier decisions about treatment and discharge, potentially shorter length of stay and fewer outpatient clinic visits.

Other benefits result from elimination of errors that arise as a result of transcription tasks in laboratories. Each transcription (for example, copying the name/number off the request form, copying the result off the analyser etc.) introduces the possibility that an error will be made: each time a transcription task is eliminated, it reduces the chance of errors occurring, ensures that information is complete, saves staff time and reduces delay. Streamlining internal laboratory procedures increases productivity and enables the laboratory to handle increased workload without increased resources.

Provision of workstations or terminals on wards and in clinics improves flexibility of access to results, as well as reducing the turnaround time further. Results can be accessible by clinical staff as soon as they are reported, eliminating the need to wait for paper copies to be delivered, or for ward and laboratory staff to transcribe details over the telephone. In addition, previous tests results for the same patient are also accessible, so that even if medical records are not to hand, nevertheless results can be found immediately.

The table below shows results from work-study measurements of the amount of time which was saved within a laboratory by using computers for routine work. The total potential saving comes to nearly 10 hours for every 100 requests.

Laboratory Time Savings

Activity	Time saved per request (minutes)
Reception and daybook entry	0.4
Production of worksheets	0.4
Result calculation	1.0
Result transcription	1.2
Creation of laboratory record	1.5
Sorting and filing	1.2
Workload statistics	0.1
Total	5.8 minutes

Other reporting services systems

Various other units provide test and investigative services similar to those provided by pathology laboratories. However, their results may not be so readily reducible to numerical data. Examples of such services include

- Microscopic anatomy (e.g. anatomical pathology, histology) whose reports describe the morphology (shape/form) and microscopic histology (cell composition) of a specimen
- Clinical imaging (e.g. radiology, ultrasound, emission tomography etc.) whose reports describe the apparent internal gross form, structure and/or activity of the body based on the images made
- Clinical physiology (e.g. electrocardiography, electroencephalography, nerve conduction, cardiac catheterisation, respiratory function etc.) whose reports describe and interpret the function of an organ or system based on complex analyses and calculations

Similar considerations as regards computerisation apply to those outlined for laboratory services above. Once again the only link between patient and test is the service accession number. In many instances there is a need to make appointments for the patient to attend for testing, a service that can readily be automated. The results are presented in the form of an electronic document.

In addition, there are reports generated by numerous referral services which provide opinions, assessments and evaluations (e.g. of speech, hearing, social environment, activities etc.), as well as reports that are prepared as a result of health events or admission (e.g. discharge notes). All of these are essentially free text material, although they may have some structured elements and any of these may be required in order to make timely and appropriate care decisions.

Report inquiry

A typical patient in hospital may have quite large numbers of tests and investigations performed both before and during their admission. The typical resident doctor in a hospital is looking after quite large numbers of patients, perhaps between 10 and 30. As a consequence he/she is likely to want to enquiry in a flexible way.

Single patient inquiries will frequently be used in order to review all aspects of that patient's status and care. These enquiries may require insertion of time limits, for example only tests related to the present admission, or falling within a specific time period may be required. Tests performed by all services may be required together, rather than requiring the user to log on to each service in sequence.

However, frequently the doctor wishes to access test results returned in the past 12, 24 or 48 hours (a period when he/she may have been off duty) for all of his/her patients. All patients are linked by the PAS to the medical staff responsible for their care, and therefore a link between any doctor and all his/her patients can be created. The capacity to review all patients in this way has been found invaluable, especially where one or more patients may be an "outlier", that is occupying a bed in another ward or a location away from the centre of that doctor's normal activities. Outliers tend to be forgotten and overlooked, to stay longer and receive less optimal care.

GP computing

General Practice is at the forefront of medical computing. The GP sector has generally been at the forefront of the use of information technology, and has consequently changed very rapidly during the past few years. Much that has happened there will have a major impact on other branches of healthcare computing.

The use of computers in general practice has grown dramatically during the period 1987–1993. The data presented here are based on the NHS GP Computing Survey covering all practices in England and Wales, April–May 1993.

Reasons for this success include:

1. During the 1970s the Department of Health sponsored an experimental computer project at Ottery St Mary near Exeter, which produced the first fully computerised "paperless" practice. This was run on a mainframe computer and provided a role-model for subsequent system developers. The Exeter software was subsequently ported to run on a microcomputer and is still on the market. An important by-product of this project was the computer prescription form which became nationally available from 1981, and enabled the spread of computer-based repeat prescribing systems

2. In 1982, as the centre-piece of its Information Technology Year (IT-82), the government launched its Micros for GPs initiative, to provide 150 practices with heavily subsidised systems. This scheme was ill-considered, but it created a great deal of political as well as professional interest in GP computing. The high profile for GP computing created at this time provided a foundation for subsequent developments

3. In 1987, two GP system suppliers launched broadly similar no-cost computer schemes, whereby any practice was provided with a computer system almost free of charge in return for agreeing to provide anonymised data about their drug prescribing, morbidity and side-effects. Each company expected to recoup its costs by selling this data to the pharmaceutical industry for post-marketing surveillance, clinical trials and market research. These schemes required sophisticated systems and every doctor needed to use a computer terminal in his or her consulting room during the consultation in order to collect the required level (95 per cent) of acute prescriptions and encounter records. This led to the

103

first widespread use of computers at the point of care. Nearly 2,000 practices (20 per cent of all practices) took up one of these schemes

4. In 1989 the Department of Health introduced direct reimbursement of some computer system costs. Fund-holding practices received up to 100 per cent reimbursement, others up to 50 per cent. Practices under the no-cost schemes were not eligible. The no-cost schemes collapsed in 1991

5. The 1990 GP Contract introduced a further financial incentive for GPs to maintain good information systems. For example, GPs now receive a substantial extra payment if they meet stringent targets for preventive medical procedures such as immunisations and screening. The combination of direct reimbursement and the demands of the new contract led to a boom in the installation of GP computer systems during 1990–91

6. In 1991, the principle of software accreditation was introduced for fund-holding software. This principle was extended to GP-FHSA links in 1993, and from 1994 all GP systems will require third-party accreditation as a precondition for reimbursement. One objective of accreditation is to bring all systems up to the same standard and to facilitate links to the FHSA, to hospitals and to community services.

Links from the practice to other parts of the NHS will be the next major growth area. The following table shows the relationship between GPs desire for links and the number of GPs with links:

GP Links to:	Desired Use	Actual Use
FHSA	79%	6%
Laboratory	78%	3%
Hospital (e.g. consultants)	75%	2%

The scale of the desire for links is put into perspective by noting that 43 per cent of computerised practices wish for more VDUs and 39 per cent more printers. Similarly the actual use of links contrasts with 29 per cent keeping full clinical records, and a further 61 per cent with partial clinical records on computer.

GP computer systems are heavily used. The average time spent using the computer each week by each user is shown below:

User	Hours/week
Receptionist	16.8
Practice Manager	13.6
GP (partner)	16.1
Practice Nurse	10.9
Secretary	15.5
Computer Staff	25.0
Fundholding Staff	25.9

Fundholding and computer staff are heavy users where they are employed.

A remarkable feature of GP computerisation in the UK is the use of systems by doctors and nurses for clinical purposes, not just by clerical staff for administrative and financial tasks. The proportion of doctors who use their computer for the following tasks is:

Medical audit	77%
Viewing clinical data in consulting room	62%
Acute prescribing in consulting room	58%
Entry of clinical data on all consultations	34%

The average number of terminals in each practice is 2.8 VDUs and 2.4 printers for single handed practices, increasing to 14.6 VDUs and 10.2 printers for those with six or more partners.
The main uses of the computer are:

Patient registration	98%
Repeat prescribing	94%
Clinical records (full or part)	90%
Call and recall	84%
Annual practice report	80%
Audit	77%
Acute prescribing	58%
Referral letters	51%
Word-processing	48%
Spreadsheets	30%
Full clinical records	29%
Protocols of care	29%
Payroll	29%
Accounts	25%
Graphics	15%
Desk-top publishing	14%
Statistics	11%

On average, computerised practices use the computer for more than ten of the tasks listed above. This figure illustrates the extensive use of software applications within computerised practices.

The level of user satisfaction with their computer systems is shown below:

Attribute	% Satisfied
Ease of use	81%
Range of facilities	72%
Back-up services	59%
Documentation	55%
Cost	44%

The picture presented above shows one of the few success stories in healthcare computing, yet it has not been without its problems. Few if any of the suppliers have made consistent profits. The reasons for this seem to be that:

1. The prices charged for systems have been low, in part because GPs need to spend their own money and have only limited funds, in part because the upper levels for reimbursement set by FHSAs are low, and in part as a consequence of fierce competition
2. The cost of sale to practices is usually high. Practices are advised to shop around and not to buy the first system they see
3. The cost of support is high. GPs and their staff are naive computer users and have no source of advice open to them other than their supplier. This means that practices make greater use of help lines and support services than is usual
4. Changes in NHS regulations such as the 1990 Contract, Fund-holding, GP-FHSA links and system accreditation have each required substantial investment in software development

This may seem of little concern to the buyers of systems, but there is a serious underlying issue. If businesses in the healthcare computing industry are unable to make profits, their accumulated expertise will be lost to other more profitable endeavours. When the buyer returns to the marketplace next, there will be fewer suppliers, less choice and no ongoing investment in product development.

Patient register

The patient register is a list of all patients registered with the practice. An accurate register is essential to check capitation payments and to provide the base figure for calculating whether the practice is reaching its targets for immunisations, smears and screening. A large part of each GPs income is based on the number of registered patients (capitation) and the percentage which meets preventive medicine targets.

Traditionally the patient register was called the age/sex register, following recommendations from the Royal College of General Practitioners during the 1960s that all practices should keep a card index sorted by age and sex to allow rapid identification of patients reaching certain ages for call and recall, and to check capitation payments. Computer-based registers allow quick retrieval and sorting by age/sex, by name, registered doctor, address or postcode.

When a new patient registers with a practice the reception staff need to inform the FHSA. The FHSA checks that this is not a duplication against their local records and at the NHS Central Registry at Stockport. Then the FHSA sends for the patient's medical record from the previous GP and forwards this to the new practice. If the patient has moved from one FHSA area to another then both FHSAs are involved. The whole process is time consuming and slow, taking up to three months for notes to arrive at the new practice. Until the notes arrive the patient must be treated without the benefit of any previous written information with all of the dangers that involves. The situation should be improved by computerisation at the NHS Central Registry, FHSA procedures and electronic GP-FHSA links.

Call and recall

The basic principle of all call and recall procedures is to identify specific groups of patients from the practice population and to ask them to attend a clinic. The organisation of efficient call and recall systems is complex, and requires good organisation as well as adequate computing facilities.

Most practices organise their call and recall on a monthly basis. For example, consider what is needed to identify and contact those eligible for cervical cytology. The first task is to identify women who are:

- Within specified age ranges
- Now due for preset call or recalls (i.e. no record of this service for past 2 years)
- Have not responded to previous letters.

In addition the program should exclude patients who:

- Have stated that they do not want to be screened
- Are not eligible for the procedure (e.g. have had a hysterectomy)
- Have already made an appointment to attend for screening
- Have already attended for screening, but whose test results are not back from the laboratory
- Who have not been given time to respond to previous letters.

The computer groups patients into categories so that each one is sent an appropriate personalised letter. The system can generate first, second and third letters if patients do not respond to the first request. At the end of each run the computer prints out a statistical report which monitors practice performance against targets.

The computer's data-base has to be kept rigorously up to date. Each letter sent out and every response from each patient has to be recorded. Each test needs to be entered and every test report must be checked by a doctor to specify appropriate action and recall period before it is recorded on the computer.

Computerised prescribing

Handwritten prescriptions are frequently illegible, creating serious problems for the pharmacist as well as risks to patient health. Computer printed scripts are clear and explicit, and the prescribing software usually includes automatic checks for known sensitivities, contra-indications and drug-drug interactions. The computer maintains a complete medication history, allowing the doctor to see at once what has happened in the past, as well as all other concurrent medications. The usage of drugs can be monitored and audited with ease.

Where prescribing software is used, formularies can be set up to list and identify the practice's preferred drugs first. This makes it easier for doctors to select low-cost (generic) items from the formulary, whilst not preventing use of non-formulary items. The use of such formularies is likely to save large sums on the drugs bill.

Computerised repeat prescribing saves a great deal of secretarial and medical time, whilst providing the practice with full control over issue, authorisation and monitoring of repeat prescriptions. Manual repeat prescribing systems require patient's notes to be pulled and updated every time a new prescription is issued, and all of the details to be transcribed — a tedious, time-consuming and error-prone chore.

Medical record fragmentation

Medical record fragmentation is a growing problem. Patients and providers of healthcare services are becoming increasingly mobile, while current approaches to care involve ever larger professional teams, requiring greater sharing of records. In many parts of the world the problem is exacerbated by the freedom of patients to choose their care service providers. This results in an uncontrolled proliferation of unconnected part records spread around the country.

Consumption of care services should not impose special restrictions on the patients, for example, in terms of restricting their freedom to travel. Care service providers should ensure that the provision of best quality care does not impose such restrictions. Providers must try to ensure continuity and integrity of care services, but there is no way of knowing when and where patients will next make contact with care services. This raises significant problems in trying to ensure that adequate information is available for consultations.

Hard copy (paper) medical records can do little to facilitate sharing of information. However, even if we had already adopted electronic medical records, the situation might be little different in terms of shared access to them. Although the part-records in each location might then be in a form that enabled them to be moved quickly and conveniently to any required location, we would still need an infrastructure that could support this process.

The best place to store information is generally where it will be of the greatest value. The location of the greatest value is clearly with the patient, since the information will be required in connection with patient care events and contacts. Hence the term Patient Held Medical Records (PHMRs). Few patients are likely to feel comfortable with the idea of carrying around bulky folders of paper records, including images. However, all the available data could be condensed into a compact form (e.g. an optical memory device) and given to the patient to carry.

It is not necessary to carry all the data on one's person. It should be sufficient just to have a synopsis of what the various record fragments contain, and a list providing an index of where they are located, as long as patients have a means of enabling their doctor (provider) of their choice to access core elements from that list at will. This could be done using a much lower capacity personal storage device, such as an integrated circuit (IC or smart) card, together with an electronic network that permits the data to be moved. Health communications networks which can provide this functionality are already being developed in many countries, providing a key part of the necessary infrastructure.

This communications process that is required is different from conventional electronic data interchange in one important way. Conventional EDI is based on the "push" concept: an individual decides to send you a message. If you want to control the process, you have to initiate it: if you need a specific set of data, you have to request that it is sent to you. When the next encounter with the health service is not anticipated by the individuals who hold the relevant data (which is the situation more often than not), the information will not be available as required.

A provider could ask for relevant details, but without knowing who holds what details, where and how they are organised and referenced, the probability of a speedy response is poor. The capacity for a provider to initiate a speedy and efficient process of information acquisition, that is of "pulling" it from its sources, is essential. This in effect *reverses* the normal flow of electronic messages — the intended recipient *initiates* the message in order to "pull" materials that he/she requires from the sender's files.

This requires:

1. A secure compact personal health synopsis, indexing what record fragments are held for a specified individual, where and by whom

2. A means of uniquely identifying and authenticating, for data protection purposes
   - The provider who is seeking access to the records, whether stored locally or remotely
   - The person to whom the records relate, and their consent to the request for access

3. A means of extracting the required data from their repository and delivering them in a readable and intelligible form to the receiver, taking into account the different ways in which they are likely to be structured and coded

4. An electronic health network that can support the necessary messaging and security, including
   - The permissions necessary for such message movements
   - Ensuring the security of data that is made accessible in this way
   - An audit trail to track who does what

Smart cards

The ideal healthcare smart card would conform to international standards that met the following criteria. First there needs to be a standard interface that would allow any standards-compliant software to read any compliant patient card. This is essential because it is not realistic to require all clinicians to use precisely the same software, nor that any card manufacturer be given a monopoly. The prototype of an open standard interface is being developed by Bull Information Systems, The University of Exeter and Abies Medical Information Systems Ltd in the European Eureka project Panacea.

The information which must be stored on the device, whatever its type and nature, would include:

- Information about the individual (e.g. identifiers, demographics, health insurance status, payer details, benefits tables)
- Information required for emergency care provision (e.g. allergies, sensitivities, chronic illnesses, life-sustaining treatments such as medications etc.)
- Recent use of care services, current medications, care plans in process etc.
- Index of care encounters, their nature and the records of them that are held, including where and by whom they are held
- Unique identifying references to the specific records (e.g. network node address, local index/reference, file structure and format etc.)

Items referenced on the card could then be selected, and a message constructed to pull them from their source. The arrangements would ensure that an audit trail is left indicating what information has been accessed in this way, when, by whom and under what authority.

Data protection

The data stored on such a device are personal and confidential: access to them must be strictly controlled and limited to those with a need to know, with the consent of the subject of the data, and, where necessary, of the holder of the records. In general the use of password by provider and cardholder will be the minimum required for access.

Opportunities for the card owner to view their own data should be made readily available. This will ensure that errors that have been made in gathering and recording the data are recognised and corrected.

There will always be the situations where a cardholder may be unable to provide the password (e.g. forgetting, unconscious) and thus be unable to provide access to the contents. This problem can be solved by providing selected professionals with the necessary "break-in" authority, consistent with the agreed privacy guidelines. To prevent abuses of this privilege, such exceptional access would be designed to generate warnings, both on the device as well as by a system-generated letter to the registered address of the subject advising of the forced access and the reasons for it.

Various suitable card-sized alternatives exist. There are:

- Optical cards, capable of storing up to 3 MBytes of data, comprising one or more areas of optical surface capable of being written/read by a laser device (just like a domestic compact disk)
- Integrated circuit cards (smart cards), comprising a computer integrated with an electronic memory; the computer limits the views of the data that are available to different authorised classes of users, providing greatly enhanced system security and flexibility of data access.

Magnetic stripe cards carry too little data (200 Bytes) to be useful, but there are other devices, such as flash memory, floppy disks and magneto-optical disks, which could be used: however, these are generally larger and/or less well suited to the task at least in their present configurations.

NHS care card

Perhaps the best known pilot study on portable medical records was the Care Card project in Exmouth in Devon, based on a smart card but without any network. In February 1989 about 9,000 patients were issued with cards supplied by Bull. The trial used 28 card readers at 13 sites and involved eight GPs in two practices, two accident and emergency units, a diabetic clinic, eight pharmacies and a large dental practice. All sites used software supplied by Abies Medical Information Systems.

The cards used in this study were restricted in capacity to 16 K bits (2 K bytes), but by using data compression techniques it was possible to store basic registration data, more than 100 dated and authenticated clinical records as well as a number of drug prescriptions on each card. The clinical records were coded using the Read Codes and included the date, author and site of origin. Space was also provided for numeric test results and free text.

The Care Card also acted as an electronic prescription. The medication records included the dosage instructions and quantity prescribed. When each prescription was dispensed, the card was updated with the date and pharmacy site.

Formal evaluation of this study and various others, particularly in France, have demonstrated that such systems can work reliably and effectively and be acceptable to both providers and patients alike. However, there are clear benefits to the use of hybrid card+network systems, as outlined above.

Issues

The development of PHMRs and networks is technically feasible. It is highly likely that they will enjoy widespread implementation in the near future. Properly implemented they could have a very positive impact on care integrity, continuity and cost containment.

However they raise some significant issues that must be explored and resolved, such as:

- Will a patient need to be able to produce their card in order to receive services at certain clinics? To do so would increase patient resistance to their introduction, and could possibly infringe their rights to appropriate care services in the event their card was mislaid
- All notes will need to be attributed to an author at the time of writing to ensure that there is no confusion as to the origin of material that has been imported from another system. Time, date, place, context and authorship will all be important in the electronic medical records
- Agreements regarding professional responsibility and compensation for errors that arise as a result of decisions taken by one individual on the basis of erroneous information provided by another will need to be reached
- Standards for the core content, structure and coding of medical records will be required to ensure that the essential content of various records produced by different systems can be read by others

Chapter 9 Coding and classification

Inaccurate or misleading information is often worse than no information at all. When information is collected by one person and used by another, both the originator and the receiver must understand it in precisely the same way. This issue may seem trivial to a reader without a knowledge of medical terminology, but in reality it is of crucial importance.

Medical terminology has developed in a relatively uncoordinated way. Many terms mean different things to different people: indeed medical records staff can often identify the institution where a doctor was trained from the way he or she uses medical terms. People use terms in the way that they and their immediate colleagues will understand; each user of a term assumes that others will understand precisely what he or she intends it to mean. There is a process of "normalisation" of terminology that takes place amongst those who share notes with each other, and common understandings are reached. In time care units may develop what amounts to their own dialect of medicine because of the ways they have chosen to use terms and the meanings they ascribe to them.

Health computing creates the potential for vastly wider sharing and reuse of information but there is an underlying assumption that each user agrees on the meaning of all of the terms used. Computers are good at manipulating symbols but do not handle the ambiguities of free text as well as human beings. It is more efficient for a computer to process data that has been reduced to numbers or codes, such as the 16-digit code on credit cards, driving licence numbers, airline reservation codes and bar codes on supermarket items. In every business where computers are widely used, almost all of the data processed are either coded or are already in an unambiguous numeric form, such as money or dates. Each sector has standardised the use of codes in that sector in order to eliminate any possibility for confusion.

Medical terminology

Unlike biology and chemistry, medical terminology lacks any formal structure. Chemical names are expressed in internationally standardised ways which uniquely describe each molecule. Every living organism has a generic and specific Latin name within a comprehensive biological taxonomy. Medical terminology has just grown through dynamic processes of linguistic development with the minimum of formalisation.

Scott Blois, in his classic work *"Information and Medicine"*, classified medical concepts into a series of levels. At the one extreme are the sub-atomic concepts which are the key to molecular biochemistry and radiation physics. At the other extreme are concepts relating to populations and societies which have an impact on health and well-being. In between are 12 levels of concepts relating to structural and functional aspects of cells, organs, body systems, whole individuals, interpersonal relationships and so on. The day-to-day vocabulary of medicine relates to almost every level in this hierarchy. Radiotherapists use subatomic particles, clinical chemists measure the concentration of molecules, haematologists study blood cells, microbiologists grow bacteria and other small organisms, radiologists review images of anatomical structures and organs, physicians are concerned with abnormal bodily functions, psychiatrists are concerned with unusual behaviour and interpersonal relationships, and epidemiologists study the spread of disease in populations. Given the scope of the domain, medical terminology is inevitably eclectic, and has adopted terms from many other sciences and disciplines.

The medical vocabulary runs to more than 100,000 words, and considerably more individual concepts. Many words in current use describe the same thing and some words are used by different groups to mean quite different things. Disagreements arise as to whether two terms are in fact synonymous, or whether there are subtle differences in meaning between them. Similarly, there are often disagreements about whether or not one term embraces the meaning of the other.

To make the situation more complicated, medicine is not only replete with synonyms (e.g. heart attack, myocardial infarction, MI, AMI, coronary thrombosis etc.), but there are also:

- *homonyms*, which are words that have more than one meaning depending upon the context (e.g. ventricle — of the heart or the brain)

- *eponyms*, where the name of a person, often the first to describe an entity, is used to refer to that entity. This adds synonyms as well as more homonyms (for example where one person, such as von Recklinghausen, described more than one entity)

- *acronyms*, which involve using the leading letter of selected words to describe an entity (e.g. MI for myocardial infarction, or mitral incompetence)

- *abbreviations*, which are short forms that are often unique to an individual, group or specialty, and may not be understood throughout the profession
- *spelling errors*, because many health professionals are poor spellers, and often even worse at accurately entering a string of characters at the keyboard.

Using human intelligence and general knowledge of the context and of medical practice, it is normally possible for one professional to correctly interpret a recorded note written by another. However, all too often even humans get it wrong.

Medicine is a domain of imprecise terminology. It is also probably the most information intensive of the professions, where decisions are made on interpretations of large and complex data sets. Further, the community has an expectation of health professionals that is less and less tolerant of errors. Add to that the need for larger numbers of professionals to participate in sharing the care of an individual, and the need for terminological precision becomes clear.

Classification

Classification is defined as the systematic placement of entities or concepts into categories which share some common attribute, quality or property. For example, biological classification places plants and animals into a hierarchical taxonomy according to similarities in structure, origin etc. that indicate a common relationship. The major biological classifications are by Kingdom, Division (plants), Phylum (animals), Class, Order, Family, Genus and Species.

Every classification has a purpose, and that purpose determines how items are grouped together into classes. For example, you can take a bowl of fruits and divide them into classes based on colour and size, or on consistency and shape, or on seed position and methods of propagation, or on shelf life and sensitivity to refrigeration depending on what it is you plan to use the classification for. Exactly the same applies in medicine, except that there are so many more different possible uses for classification systems. Hence the large number of medical classification systems in existence.

Any attempt to produce a single universal classification for every possible purpose in medicine is doomed. Any set of objects can be classified in an almost unlimited number of ways for an unlimited number of purposes.

Attempts to use a classification for purposes other than those for which it was designed are likely to cause unpredictable problems. In practice some classifications have proven useful for applications for which they were not originally intended. For example, the International Classification of Diseases (ICD) was originally designed to record mortality statistics, but it is now widely used to record acute hospital activity (though not without criticism).

Coding

A code is defined as a sequence of symbols, most often letters or digits, serving to designate an object or concept and used for identification or selection purposes. A code is simply an alternative way of naming an entity or concept. Some codes are selected for their ease of handling by computers, whilst in the past others have been selected because they are meaningful to humans.

A code can be made up of any symbols or characters. Typically, codes use the alphanumeric characters on a standard keyboard, but any other characters and marks that can be recognised by the computer are quite acceptable in codes.

Codes may be assigned to entities in an ordered way or at random. Ordered coding systems may be hierarchical or non-hierarchical. The advantage of an ordered coding system, and especially of an hierarchical system, is that it makes manipulations of the coded data much easier.

Consider the differences between:

system 1 (random)		system 2 (ordered and hierarchical)	
code	meaning	code	meaning
AMI	acute myocardial infarct	G	cardiovascular diagnosis
OMI	old myocardial infarct	G3	cardiac diagnosis
MI	myocardial infarct	G30	acute myocardial infarction
PHA	posterior heart attack	G300	acute anterior infarct
IHA	inferior heart attack	G301	acute anterolateral infarct
AHA	anterior heart attack	G302	acute anteroseptal infarct
		G303	acute septal infarct
			.... etc

System 1 would be more easily used by humans, who could recognise and assign codes, since each code is intrinsically meaningful (although you would soon run out of unique 3–character codes). And either system could be used to find instances of, for example, *acute myocardial infarction* as a generic entity (search for AMI in system 1; G30 in system 2). However, to summarise the data for **all** acute myocardial infarct diagnoses would be difficult in system 1, where the search would need to be set up for AMI or MI or PHA or IHA or AHA, whilst in system 2 it would be much easier to search for all codes starting with the characters G30.

Consider also the problems of exchanging data between systems using each of these coding systems. Whilst both of these systems may work well enough for manipulation of their own data, it is immediately apparent that exchange of data between the two systems would be difficult, since the entities in one classification do not map directly to corresponding entities in the other. This, then, defeats one of the objects of classification and coding of the data, if the data cannot readily be reused for all the required purposes.

The scope of any computer application is ultimately constrained by the scope of the coding systems employed. Comprehensive sets of codes need to be provided, covering all of the concepts and terms which might be used by the application. Coding systems need to be comprehensive in breadth and depth of cover. For example, a drug coding system would be clearly unacceptable if many drugs were omitted.

Medical knowledge and terminology is growing all the time and it is essential that any coding scheme incorporates the necessary flexibility to enable unpredictable future developments and expansion. Codes must never be reused or redefined to mean something different from one version to another (backwards compatibility).

Every classification and coding system comprises three fundamental components:

1. a preferred text descriptor for each entity in natural language
2. codes which are alternate names for each entity. The preferred text descriptor and its corresponding code are true synonyms, that is, they mean exactly the same. For example ICD-9 code 413 means *angina pectoris*
3. indexation systems and navigation tools that enable a user to locate the required term and code

It is a common mistake to confuse coding with classification. The error arises because each category within a classification is usually allocated a code number and the process of classification requires codes to be entered onto a form or a computer terminal. Codes can refer to both unclassified objects and concepts as well as to classes and groupings. Anything can be given a code — remember, a code is just an alternative name for something: a classification system is not necessary for entities to be assigned codes.

Classifications — for whom and what for?

Few clinical users of health information systems display any intrinsic interest in classifications or codes. On the other hand, everyone involved in data manipulation and analysis is totally absorbed by them. Codes are needed for **computer** processing, but text descriptors are what **people** understand. Well-designed programs used for data entry often hide all codes from users. Doctors and nurses naturally want to record information in the form, language and detail that is of greatest benefit to them in the context of reaching decisions about individual patients. On the one hand clinical notes require comprehensive detail about individual patients, but on the other hand statistical analysis needs entities to be grouped into a relatively small number of discrete categories, submerging much of the finer detail.

The conflicting requirements of clinical records and statistical applications can be reconciled by using hierarchical structures. A hierarchical coding scheme can be thought of as an inverted tree with its trunk or root at the top. Each item consists of a code with a structure which specifies its position relative to all other codes.

The structure of the code increases in detail from left to right, with the first character of the code specifying the main section of the classification, the second giving greater specificity and so on. System 2 in the example above is an example of a hierarchical classification.

Other relevant definitions

A **nomenclature** is a list of approved terms used in a technical area. A comprehensive nomenclature for the whole of biomedicine may need to be very large.

A **thesaurus** provides a way of linking together terms which are conceptually related to help the user find the precise term required. Roget's Thesaurus is a well-known example, and many word processors also incorporate thesauri.

A **glossary** provides a definition of each term or phrase. Detailed unambiguous definitions (in addition to the preferred term) are essential when the precise meaning of a code and term is not crystal clear. Some classifications provide detailed definitions of the criteria whereby an entity may be included in or excluded from a specific class.

Taxonomy is the systematic placement of things or concepts into a hierarchical (tree-like) classification.

A **dictionary** is a volume which contains the words of a language, arranged in alphabetical order, with their meanings or definitions, pronunciation and derivation or origin.

International Classification of Disease

The International Classification of Disease (ICD) is at present in its 9th revision (ICD9, released 1975) and is available in an extended form with additional clinical modifications (ICD9CM). ICD is developed and maintained under the auspices of the World Health Organisation. Most governments, including the UK, have agreed with the WHO to collect national statistics using the ICD-9, and to move to ICD-10 on April 1st, 1995.

ICD was initially developed as a means of comparing the causes of death between countries. However, it has become widely used as a basis for morbidity returns from acute hospitals.

There are 21 chapters of ICD10, each of which relates to an organ system of the body. Within each chapter the various disease entities are listed as 3-digit codes, with an optional fourth and fifth digit for additional detail. The chapters are:

1. Infectious and parasitic diseases   A00–B99
2. Neoplasms   C00–D48
3. Diseases of blood and blood forming organs and certain disorders involving the immune mechanism   D50–D89
4. Endocrine, nutritional and metabolic diseases   E00–E90

5. Mental and behavioural disorders   F00–F99
6. Diseases of the Nervous system   G00–G99
7. Diseases of the eye and adnexa   H00–H59
8. Diseases of the ear and mastoid process   H60–H95
9. Diseases of the Circulatory system   I00–I99
10. Diseases of the Respiratory system   J00–J99
11. Diseases of the Digestive system   K00–K93
12. Diseases of Skin and subcutaneous tissue   L00–L99
13. Diseases of musculo-skeletal system and connective tissue   M00–M99
14. Diseases of the Genitourinary system   N00–N99
15. Pregnancy, childbirth and puerperium   O00–O99
16. Certain conditions originating in the perinatal period   P00–P96
17. Congenital anomalies   Q00–Q99
18. Symptoms, signs and abnormal clinical and laboratory findings not classified elsewhere   R00–R99
19. Injury, poisoning and other consequences of external factors   S00–T98
20. External causes of mobidity and mortality   V01–Y98
21. Factors influencing health status and contact with health services   Z00–Z99

Taking this a little further, chapter 10 (diseases of the respiratory system) subdivides into:

acute upper respiratory infections	J00–J06
influenze and pneumonia	J10–J18
other acute lower respiratory infections	J20–J22
other diseases of the upper respiratory tract	J30–J39
chronic lower respiratory diseases	J40–J47
lung disease due to external agents	J60–J70
other respiratory diseases principally affecting the interstituin	J80–J84
Suppurative and necrotic conditions of the lower respiratory tract	J85–J86
other diseases of pleura	J90–J94
other diseases of the respiratory system	J95–J99

Going to one further level of detail, acute respiratory infections are divided into:

J00 acute nasopharyngitis (common cold)
J01 acute sinusitis
J02 acute pharyngitis
J03 acute tonsillitis
J04 acute laryngitis and tracheitis
J05 acute obstructive laryngitis [croup] and epiglottitis
J06 acute upper respiratory infections of multiple and unspecified sites

Each of these may be further subdivided with one additional digit added. Disease entities are typically represented in the form J04.1 (acute tracheitis).

A further section provides codes for the morphology of neoplasms in a slightly different format (e.g. M8090/1—based cell tumour).

The language of ICD clearly indicates that it is intended for use by coders who are not directly associated with the patient and are working from notes made by the providers. The content of ICD is generally perceived as being inadequate to record the clinical detail required by hospital specialists, and inappropriate to the needs of general practitioners, community care services, long stay facilities and some other categories. Its usefulness is in being able to summarise and compare acute hospital caseloads.

Diagnosis Related Groups (DRGs) and Healthcare Resource Groups (HRG)

ICD can say something about what illnesses a specific patient may have been treated for, but this does not provide much of an insight into how serious the problem was, nor how much time, effort and resources may have been consumed in coping with it. This is where DRGs and HRGs have been found useful. The usefulness of resource consumption groupings in contract management is discussed in chapter 7.

There are several variants of resource groupers. The general arrangement of DRGs for example, is that there are 23 chapters, called major diagnostic categories (MDC) based on a body organ system in the same way as ICD or a clinical specialty. Each MDC is divided into two subsections, dependent upon whether a surgical procedure was involved: patients undergoing an operating theatre procedure directly related to the principal diagnosis during that hospitalisation are categorised as surgical. Medical groups are then further divided according to primary diagnosis, age and presence of complications and/or co-morbidities (CC) which are likely to have a significant impact on the length of hospitalisation and/or the complexity of the care required. Similarly, surgical groups are divided by type of operation, age, complications and/or co-morbidities and presence of malignancy.

Patients within the same group are likely to stay for similar lengths of time in hospital and to require equivalent complexity of care. In other words, statistically they will consume a broadly similar profile of hospital resources (iso-resource). There are a growing number of refinements of the resource grouping structure. Some have identified the need for expansions of specific areas (e.g. radiotherapy, paediatrics). Others, such as Refined DRGs (RDRGs), explicitly take account of the impact of different secondary diagnoses and complications. All systems have a process of annual review, and significant changes in groupings occur from one year to the next.

The Read Codes

The Read Codes are a structured hierarchy of medical terms, designed for use by clinicians in day-to-day patient care. The Read Codes are a super-set of other major coding and classification systems (e.g. ICD-9 and OPCS-4) and have been cross-mapped to those codes. Such links are vital for use in national and international comparisons.

The development of the Read Codes began in 1983 as a joint effort by James Read, a GP in Loughborough, and Abies Informatics Ltd. In April 1990 the Read Codes were purchased by the Secretary of State for Health and are now Crown Copyright. The Department of Health has established the NHS Centre for Coding and Classification (with Dr James Read as its first director) to develop and maintain the codes. The Read Codes are being improved continuously and upgrades are issued quarterly. The first version of the Read Codes with 30-character terms was completed in 1986. This format is known as Version 1. Version 2 provides alternative 60- and 192-character terms, and became available in 1991. Version 3 became available in 1994 (see below).

The Read Codes were developed specifically for use with computers (no paper version has ever been published) to enable fast data entry needing no typing skills, for exchange of data between computers, and for ease of information retrieval. The codes have been kept short (5 characters) for reasons of efficiency, and for ease of use they comprise printable characters (numerals 0–9, letters A–Z and a–z) which can be interpreted by users and software developers alike. The use of codes with both upper and lower case letters as well as numerals (but excluding the letters O and I, which might be confused with numerals 0 and 1) gives 58 options at each node. Hence, 5-character codes could accommodate up to 656,356,768 entities.

The Read Codes provide the most comprehensive clinical coding system in widespread use anywhere. In April 1994, the use of the Read Codes became a condition for accreditation (and hence reimbursement) of all GP systems in England, Wales and Scotland. Currently there are about 100,000 preferred terms and a further 150,000 synonyms or index terms. The Read Codes cover the whole breadth of clinical medicine from subjective and objective findings, diagnoses, procedures and treatment, to administrative arrangements, all using the form and language which clinicians normally use.

Specifically the Read Codes have separate sections for:

- diseases, based on ICD
- surgical procedures and operations, based on OPCS-4
- drugs, based on the British National Formulary
- history, symptoms, family history, past medical history and social history

- examination and signs, organised by body system
- tests, measurements, laboratory investigations and results
- other therapy and therapeutic procedures
- imaging and other diagnostic procedures
- preventive medical care and patient education
- occupations and occupational risk factors
- administration

The Read Codes have a five-level hierarchy with up to 60 items under each node, providing increasing fineness of granularity, e.g.:

- level 1   infectious disease
- level 2   viral disease with exanthemata
- level 3   rubella
- level 4   rubella with neurological complications
- level 5   rubella encephalomyelitis

The text descriptors (rubrics) are clearly understandable on their own and are of limited length. Three versions are provided, one with 30-character rubrics, the second using up to 60 characters, and the third allowing up to 192 characters. On conventional 80-column screens, 60 characters is perhaps the maximum length for any single line of text, while still providing sufficient space for a date field, an indicator of the author and perhaps a couple of extra fields. Fixed length rubrics help programmers to set aside specific areas when designing computer displays and reports.

In summary the key features of the Read Codes are:

- designed solely for use with computers. No paper version has ever been published
- developed by practising doctors, for use by practising doctors
- comprehensive in scope, covering diagnoses, medication, operations, history, examination, investigations and administrative procedures
- compatible with and cross-mapped to national statistical requirements (ICD-9, ICD-10 and OPCS-4)
- hierarchical alphanumeric structure with 5 levels and 60 possibilities at each node, giving a total code space of more than 600,000,000 options
- continuous development, on the basis that medical development will never stop, with regular updates
- simple hierarchical structure (taxonomy) that simplifies software development and integration into applications

The simple hierarchical structure of the original Read Codes[1] has a fundamental problem in that the code value is used both as a unique identifier and as a means of ordering a list of terms for display purposes. This creates problems whenever it becomes necessary to add additional terms into the classification or to change the order of display lists. For example, the introduction of ICD-10 involves significant changes from ICD-9. The solution is to separate functions of unique identification of medical concepts and terms (the proper job of a code value), and that of display hierarchy (the proper role of classification and taxonomy).

Version 3 of the Read Codes incorporates these changes and was completed in April 1994. However, separation of identifying and hierarchical functions of the Read Codes has made greater demands of software implementations and navigation tool requirements.

International Classification of Primary Care (ICPC)

ICPC is a system designed for use in primary care, and was developed under the auspices of the World Organisation of National Colleges, Academies and Academic Associations of General Practitioners/Family Physicians (WONCA). It is based on a model of an episode of illness, which may comprise one or more health care encounters, all related to the same problem.

It has a biaxial structure, with 17 body organs or systems represented on one axis (chapters), and 7 components of the clinical encounter on the other. These are:

Chapters:
- A – General and unspecific
- B – Blood and blood forming organs
- D – Digestive
- F – Eye
- H – Ear, hearing
- K – Circulatory
- L – Musculoskeletal, locomotor
- N – Neurological
- P – Psychological
- R – Respiratory
- S – Skin
- T – Endocrine, metabolic and nutritional
- U – Urological
- W – Pregnancy, child-bearing and family planning
- X – Female genital and breasts
- Y – Male genital
- Z – Social

Components of the encounter are divided into three headers, the second of which has five subsections. To the right of each component section below are the codes for use within that section.

Reasons for Encounter:
1 – Symptoms and complaints   (01–29)

Encounter Processes:
2 – Diagnostic, screening and preventive procedures   (30–49)
3 – Treatment procedures and medications   (50–59)
4 – Test results   (60–61)
5 – Administrative   (62)
6 – Referral and other reasons for encounter   (63–69)
Diagnosis:
7 – Diagnoses and disease entities   (70–99)

An ICPC record code is written in the form of an upper case letter (for the chapter) followed by two numerals, for example:

H01 (meaning complaint of earache).
W15 (meaning complaint of infertility)
X87 (meaning uterovaginal prolapse)

Coding system comparison

The following table shows a breakdown of the number of codes and classes in some widely used coding systems and classifications. This table demonstrates the comprehensive scope of the Read Codes, and the difficulty of making any valid comparison of the Read Codes with classifications such as the Anatomical Therapeutic Classification (ATC) for drugs and the International Classification of Primary Care (ICPC), which are widely used in Europe.

The version of the Read Codes shown is the so-called unified set which uses 5-character codes for diagnosis and surgical procedures and 4-character codes elsewhere.

CLASSIFICATION	DISEASES	PROCEDURES	DRUGS	OTHER	TOTAL
ICD-9 CM	12,943	3,735	—		16,678
READ V2	27,522	8,591	13,371	12,283	61,767
OPCS-4	7,858	—		—	7,858
ATC	—	—	1,043	—	1,043
ICPC	719	—	—	—	719

Registration of coding schemes

While a single standard comprehensive international coding system would seem to be the ideal solution this may not be practical. For instance, codes are used to identify objects such as hospitals, staff, patients, machines and products, as well as medical concepts such as diseases, treatments and tests. Many coding systems already exist and have already been adopted for specific purposes. These arrangements cannot easily be changed.

The proposed solution to this problem, which is the subject of the first European Standard in healthcare computing (ENV 1068: 1993), is to set up an international registration scheme, under the aegis of the

World Health Organisation (WHO), to provide all healthcare coding schemes with an unique identifier, or Healthcare Coding scheme Designator (HCD). This register provides a six-character designator for each coding scheme, together with precise information about the procedures used for supplying and updating the codes in electronic form.

One important rule for any registered coding scheme is that when upgrades are produced, additional codes may be added as new versions are developed, but none of the meanings of any existing codes should change. If codes need to be reallocated, then a new registration identifier must be applied for and issued. This rule applies to all types of codes and identifiers, including those used for people, places, objects, manufactured articles, computer databases and medical terms.

Registered coding schemes will be used in messages in the following way. Whenever a computer sends a message to another system, for example from a hospital to a GP, it will need to specify what coding schemes it is using. If the receiving system recognises the identifiers, the message will be accepted, otherwise it will be refused. The registration scheme allows any coding scheme to be used, but market forces will determine which are most successful. Software developers will minimise the number of coding schemes they support.

Chapter 10 Electronic communications

There is no technical barrier to communication of health information between systems large or small, local or remote. Experience in other sectors indicates that major improvements in efficiency and productivity can be achieved by moving information faster and sharing it between a larger number of individuals.

Many developments have been undertaken for specific health information communication needs, for example to exchange data between provider and laboratories, between community and hospital doctors, and between providers and administrative agencies and purchasers. In 1993 New Zealand launched the first national health information network offering a point of connection to every authorised health sector agency and individual, aimed at providing a highway for the exchange of all types of health-related information. The UK NHS intends to achieve a similar penetration in 1995.

Every home, practice and hospital computer has the inherent potential to share information with any other computer, to link in to all sorts of systems and to make use of their resources. At present most computers are "stand-alone" but each could readily become a node in a network, or be linked to many different servers of software and information. Laboratory results, orders, messages, information, pictures, claims and other information can be exchanged with other care providers and services, with local hospitals, with insurers and third party payers. We could retrieve information from a wide range of bibliographic systems, or interact with electronic shopping guides, stockbroking or financial services.

Effective electronic communication relies upon a complex infra-structure of standards and conventions. Almost everyone who has ever owned a computer will have experienced the frustration of discovering that they could not quickly and easily establish links with other computers (e.g. their local pathology service), or with a network service or even to a particular printer or other device (e.g. MODEM) they may have acquired.

The basis of communication

The requirements for any effective and error-free communication are indeed complex. People often ignore them, and as a consequence human communications are fraught with errors and misunderstandings. All too often a simple communication error lies at the root of a human dispute or misadventure. Think of telephone conversations when we call the wrong number and talk to complete strangers, talk over each other, missing or misunderstanding words and so on.

Humans can usually extract the content of a message and interpret it in the context of general knowledge of the world as well as specific knowledge of healthcare and of the context to which the message refers. We can read between the lines, fill in missing data and draw inferences from what is and is not contained in the message to reach interpretations and conclusions, which go beyond the information communicated, and may be even be false. Computers are much worse at coping with the uncertainties and problems that arise because they lack "common sense" and the basic intelligence that we use to make sense of a message, even when it is poorly constructed and partially scrambled. Computers cannot tolerate any sort of ambiguity, and are unable to make sense of a message unless it conforms exactly with a predefined set of rules and standards.

In computer communications nothing can be left to chance. Rules, formats, templates and protocols have to be developed for each and every type of message, and for every aspect of the electronic transmission from one machine to another. Sophisticated communications environments can establish a secure data link, transmit data, detect and take corrective action for any transmission errors, order segments to be retransmitted, acknowledge and even respond automatically to the content of the message, and then reset themselves in readiness for the next message to be transmitted. Perhaps it's a pity we humans do not emulate this desirable state of affairs in our own communications!

Making messages meaningful

The objective of Electronic Data Interchange (EDI) is to transmit a message between computers at the sender and receiver ends in such a way that the message is complete, unambiguous and error-free, and conveys the same meaning to the receiver as was intended by the sender. To do this, requires that the parties:

1. share a common dictionary (terms and meanings)
2. share an agreed syntax (arrangement of words)
3. agree on a mode and medium of communication (e.g. phone/fax)
4. agree on a "protocol" for communication (e.g. who speaks when, what to do if two or more speak at once, how to deal with line faults and errors)

The need for each of these is relatively self-explanatory. The need for a common **dictionary** (a set of terms with a set of definitions of those terms) is an absolute prerequisite of any attempt to communicate, since unless words mean the same to sender and receiver, accurate communication is impossible. This is one of the areas where medicine runs into problems immediately, since there is considerable disagreement between health professionals both about terminology and the precise meaning and implications of selected terms.

The need for an agreed **syntax** also raises problems. The precise juxtaposition of words, and the placement of punctuation can radically affect the meaning of a sentence. However, the "natural language" that most people speak and write tends to ignore many of the rules of syntax and relies for its meaning on physical expression, non-verbal signals, the general context and on the specialised and common knowledge of the communicators, who may often speak in what amounts to "shorthand", especially where they share the same specialty.

The need for agreement on the **mode** and **medium** of the message arises because electronic messages can be sent in so many different ways. The data from one computer may be compressed, encrypted, segmented into packets, passed through switches and routed across various different networks, frequency modulated onto a microwave beam and bounced off a satellite on its way to the destination.

In general terms there must be:

- a conducting pathway providing an end-to-end physical link between sender and receiver which transfers the bits from origin to destination: this may involve routing the signal appropriately across various media and networks, each of which may have its own rules and regulations regarding the packaging, addressing, charging for and handling of the message (just like different postal services)
- rules to deal with the various problems that may arise between source and destination: rules for how to initiate and terminate a contact or session, to prevent or manage the situation when two data streams collide, to re-establish a link when there is a line failure, to accommodate for noise on the line, and so on

In many formal environments, such as Parliament, or committee meetings, there are well established rules on "protocol", for example, the speaker may need to hold a "token" in order to be able to address the group; and interruptions are not allowed until the present speaker has finished. Exactly the same sort of rules are used in computer communications protocols.

Electronic communications

Electronic messages require all the same conventions as humans for interaction, and some more. Where computers are linked together in any way, each terminal is called a **node**. Nodes can send and receive messages, so each node has a unique identifier or **address** which identifies where this computer can be found and therefore how to send messages to it. Every user of a network has their own unique **identifier** which means that the system can recognise them and ensure that they have access to the appropriate files and resources, no matter which physical terminal they are using. The term **network** or **node-user address (NUA)** is often used to refer to the combination of physical node and its current user. The NUA remains fixed only for the duration of the current **session** of connection between that node and the network to which it is linked.

Communications can be set up on the basis of "batch" or "interactive" messaging. In the batch mode, a message is sent, and all the sender gets is an acknowledgment (or error message) to indicate that the message has reached the intended destination. Interactive messaging, however, is more like a discussion: sending a message can elicit an automatic reply from the receiver, and this can in its turn initiate further messages from sender and receiver. For example, if a user wished to look up a person in a master patient index, an interactive session would be required. If, on the other hand, the task was simply to send mail, a batch session would be quite sufficient.

Networks and systems

It is clear that computer users require access to wide area communications, whether for the purpose of exchanging messages, collecting laboratory results, keeping in touch with the literature, or manipulating money matters. It is essential that everyone who makes use of the technology has some understanding of the broad underpinning concepts. This section has been designed to introduce most of the "buzz words" in communications and explain simply what they are and where they fit into the grand scheme. Inevitably many have been left out too, since this is not designed to be a reference work in communications.

Every file or command can be represented as a stream of data, large or small. The data stream can be either **analogue** or **digital.** Digital data streams are the most commonly used in modern equipment: the information is reduced to a series of **bits,** or **binary digits.** Digital data moving along a wire appears as a sequence of voltage pulses, all of the same size and duration and regularly spaced. It is the pattern of the bits which carries the information. By contrast, analogue data streams are based on incremental or proportional representation: analogue data moving along a wire appears as a succession of changes in the voltage, or alternatively as a succession of tones of different frequencies.

If the data network is based on digital technology, any analogue data (such as from an older type of telephone) will need to be converted into digital form using an analogue to digital (A to D) converter. Conversely if the data stream is digital (e.g. from a computer) but the network is analogue (e.g. most existing telephone networks), the data must be converted into analogue form by a D to A converter. Typically this function is carried out using a MODEM (Modulator demodulator) unit, which converts the digits into tones or notes of different frequency. A second MODEM at the other end converts the data back to digital form for the receiving computer.

Digital networks can only carry digital data streams: analogue networks require analogue streams. The technologies are totally different, but converters exist to link the two together as required. The advantage of digital over analogue signals is the potential for higher transmission speeds, logical control protocols, multimedia transmissions and error detection and checking. Hence the present emphasis on replacing existing telephone circuits with high speed digital networks based on broadband optical fibre technology, explained in more detail below.

Let us now look in more detail at the technology that is used to move the messages around a network.

Networks

There are just three ways of moving information from one place to another.

The first is to move it physically, usually on paper but possibly on electronic media, such as tape, diskette or card. Conventional paper records can be transferred from one doctor to another — even in different specialties — simply by handing them over. Such transfers, referrals and requests for second opinions happen all the time. The capacity for easy exchange and sharing of clinical data between specialists, and between hospital and general practice is of growing importance in order to ensure continuity and integrity of care for individuals, as well as to improve cost-effectiveness.

The second method is to transmit information as electrical signals along a wire, as in telephone and cable networks. Most computer networks are hard-wired, and require a point-to-point connection to be in place before any communication is possible. Such cables are inflexible and expensive.

The third approach is to use wireless communication, as pioneered by portable telephones and now implemented in wireless networks. The use of wireless terminals for collection and display of patient data offers a potential solution to some of the constraints on flexibility that are imposed by the need to use fixed and hard-wired points of connection into a system.

Networks are often linked together: the Internet (IN) is a global network of thousands of computers which enable messages to be sent between almost everyone who has a link into any of the computers of networks involved.

Physical links

At the most basic level, the stream of data has to travel along some conducting medium from one computer to another. Different media have different capacities for carrying data, this being defined as their **bandwidth** and described in terms of KBits/second (KBaud). The conventional "twisted pair" of copper wires (as in the older parts of the telephone system) has a relatively narrow bandwidth, but it is possible to make better use of it by **multiplexing.**

Twisted pair cables are subject to electrical interference, since they act a bit like a radio aerial and pick-up noise from around them. However the interference may be "screened" by surrounding the conductor(s) with an earthed shield. This is called coaxial (coax) or screened cable. Screening extends the useful bandwidth of the copper cable.

Modern communications requires ever wider bandwidths for higher speed communications (e.g. image transmission), so that more bits can be sent over the same physical conductors at faster rates. Thus **optical fibres** and **microwave** (radio) linkages are now widely used. The former uses light as the "carrier" and modulates signals onto beams of coherent (laser-generated) light which are then passed along a fibre or fibre bundle made of glass. Optical fibres are flexible and durable, and can carry data on an almost unlimited number of simultaneous channels (multiplexing) by the use of various different light frequencies. Microwave transmission makes use of normal radio transmission techniques, modulating signals onto radio waves.

Multiplexing involves sending several signals simultaneously over the same transmission medium. Each signal is **modulated** around a different base frequency, just like radio signals on the airwaves. The data carried can be analogue or digital in form.

Routing and message handling

Now, think of the issue of routing. In a point-to-point telephone link up, the operator makes a direct connection between the two nodes: the message sent by one is passed through switches which ensure that it goes direct to the other. This is an example of "connection-oriented" communications: the sender knows that the link is working because of the responses of the receiver. Such networks provide services to support error-free communications that connectionless networks cannot as the receiver is always directly linked in connection-oriented communication.

A connectionless network is where there is no end-to-end session between sender and receiver. Think of dropping a letter in the mail box: you have no connection with the receiver, but expect your mail to reach them because of the addressing. However you do not know when or if it arrives. The concept of mailboxes is widely used in electronic systems: if a node is temporarily off-line, the messages are put into their mailbox for them to pick up later. The mailbox is logically connected to that user ID, but may be physically located anywhere on an available network filestore.

Many message handling systems work best if the size of the message is predetermined. Larger messages are split up into small fixed size **packets.** Packets from multiple messages are all mixed in together to form a continuous stream of data: the packets each have a header to identify their destination. Fast operating switches are used to separate out and route packets to each specific destination, hence the name **packet switched** networks. Imagine a very long message (e.g. an image file): this might have to be segmented into a very large number of smaller packets for sending. Each packet may be forwarded along a different route, depending on the levels of activity and congestion on the network. In this case there must be some notation within the packets that allows the receiving station to reassemble the pieces in the correct order.

Open systems

It is frequently necessary to achieve some degree of **"interoperability"** between systems. In other words one system will be able to make remote calls on another system to perform a particular function.

We all know that it is hard enough even to share floppy disks, because there are fundamental differences between unlike machines from different stables and running under different operating systems. In fact the applications software is an extension of this problem, since much of the application relies on specific features of a specific operating system for its functionality. It is for this reason that software developed for one system cannot normally be run on another without extensive modification.

This issue is addressed by the Open Systems Interconnection (OSI) suite of standards. The goal of OSI is to enable this connectivity between machines. Open Systems compliance provides users with computer solutions that are, at least in principle, **portable, scalable** and **interoperable** between hardware provided by different manu-facturers.

Portability: for many years the computer industry has been dominated by proprietary solutions which locked purchasers into using tools provided by a single supplier. Open systems enable users to transfer data and software from hardware provided by one manufacturer to that supplied by another, providing a migration route for users to take advantage of new hardware developments.

Scalability: at one time the computer market was divided into sectors for mainframes, minicomputers and microcomputers, each using different types of software. Scalable applications run on all sizes of hardware from PCs to mainframes, allowing common software to be used throughout the organisation.

Interoperability: No hospital can hope to run all of its activities on a single computer. Data needs to be transferred between many computers. Interoperability enables easy and reliable communication between hardware supplied by different manufacturers.

In practice, the phrase "Open Systems" normally refers to computer hardware that uses a UNIX-based operating system that conforms to the POSIX (P1003.1) standard. POSIX (Portable Operating System Interface) defines interfaces to a common set of functions and services to be provided by a computer operating system. Most versions of UNIX are POSIX conformant. However POSIX is also supported by a number of other operating systems including Microsoft Windows NT and Apple Mac AUX.

The OSI model

The OSI model has seven layers: the four "lower" layers (1–4) provide for interconnection and deal with the transmission of bits from origin to destination, whilst the three "upper" layers (5–7) permit interworking of systems. Thus the "level" to which a system or network is OSI compliant determines its intrinsic capacity to support communication and interworking between systems.

The OSI layers are:

1. physical — provides the linkage to the medium that is used for sending and receiving the data (e.g. optical fibre, coaxial cable etc.): the data is actually exchanged between machines at this layer level
2. data-link — transmission of streams of data between one node and the next within a network, with capacity for limited error detection and correction
3. network — deals with the issues of routing streams of bits between networks
4. transport — provides for transmission of data to a defined quality (error detection and correction) from one point to another across whatever routes and links are involved
5. session — concerning data flow structures, distinguishing logical activities and permitting resynchronisation of links where necessary
6. presentation — concerning syntax, symbols and alphabet of information transfer
7. application — concerning semantics of information transfer

When data is transferred between machines using the OSI model, it is passed "down" from the application layer (7) on machine 1, through each successive layer (6–5–4–3–2–1), then transmitted across the link to machine 2, where it passes back "up" through levels 1–2–3–4–5–6–7 and is then actioned within the application running there. The "down" movement of data involves each successive layer putting the data from the layer above into an envelope, so data from level 7 will have 7 successive wrappers around it before it is moved through level 1 to another system. The "up" movement of data involves successively stripping off those envelopes according to the parameters of the receiving station.

The OSI model endeavours to embrace every possibility and option. Consequently the full OSI specification contains tens of thousands of alternatives and options. There are many communications protocols that are based on OSI, including the widely referred to X.25 and X.400/X.500. X.25 is the most widely implemented protocol in OSI compliant public networks, and provides support for the lower 4 OSI layers, that is up to and including the establishment of a session layer. The upper layers have to be provided by other protocols, for example message handling (X.400) and directory services (X.500).

In addition, various major users have defined their own selection of communications options, and this has led to defined OSI Profiles, such as the Government OSI Profile (**GOSIP**). This is done on the basis that few users will have the skills to be able to define appropriate profiles for themselves.

Verification and detection/ prevention of errors

In any electronic network, and especially where health messages are concerned, it is important to be able to verify that the message was received as sent, in its entirety. A variety of error detection techniques are used for this, including checks on the numbers of digits, their "**sum**" (checksum) and various other parameters. Depending on the level of error detection used in a particular communication, both sending and receiving station can be almost certain the message was received as sent. Error detection techniques may make messages slightly longer than they would otherwise be, and involve signals sent in the reverse direction to confirm the message reception.

It is always important to ensure that electronic messages do not get scrambled together. Only one node in a particular sector can be transmitting a message at a time. Nodes must be able to sense when there is a lull in traffic and inject their message. Various protocols exist to manage this problem: most well known are probably the use of **tokens** and **slots**. The tokens circulate round the network, and a node can only transmit when it captures a token: the token is reinserted into the network after the message is sent to be captured by the next mode wishing to transmit. Slots differ in that they offer fixed size "spaces" that any node can catch and fill with a packet of message.

A third major protocol permits any node to transmit whenever it senses a lull in network traffic. The more nodes there are in a network, the greater the possibility of two nodes sensing the same lull and commencing transmission simultaneously. Thus a collision detection facility must be included. This recognises that there has been a collision, terminates both messages and enforces a short time delay (which differs for each node to prevent a recurrence of the same collision) before either can transmit again: this is known as "Carrier Sense, Multiple Access, Collision Detect" or CSMA/CD. The **Ethernet** system is based on CSMA/CD protocols.

Linking networks

Often networks using different protocols and/or messages must be linked. Certain aspects of a message may be specific to the originating network, and these may need to be modified as the message is passed on in order for each network to be able to read, for example, the destination.

Messages are put into envelopes (with a header and trailer) for moving. The envelope is often specific to the network through which the message is being passed. As it passes from one network onto the next, a **bridge** is normally required to remove the message from one envelope and place it in the next. Where more than just the envelope must be changed, for example the parts of the message must be translated or reorganised in some way, a **gateway** or **router** is used.

When a large computer is linked in to a communications environment, the management of the connection protocols for the communications are often off-loaded onto a specialised **front-end processor** which acts as the interface to the network. This can handle protocol conversions, error detection and requests to resend, identification of messages that are invalid for example due to incompleteness, or parameters that fall outside the range of valid values, and so on. The front-end processor can deal with all this whilst the main processor continues its normal tasks without interruptions.

Some other common communications environments

There are a range of communications protocols that pertain principally to the telephone system: however these are of considerable importance since much of the digital data to be exchanged must flow over telephone links. These protocols are standardised by Comité Consultatif International Telegraphique et Telephonique (CCITT) the body responsible for the development of international telecommunications standards.

The standards for MODEM links define importantly the maximum speed of data exchange that can be supported and are prefixed with the letter 'V'. These are typically in the 4,800 — 9,600 Baud range (e.g. V.27/V.32), but faster MODEMs can run at 14.4 or 19.2 KBaud, and devices running at up to 48KBaud are available (e.g. V.35).

Newer phone exchanges are being built to a new communications protocol called ISDN (Integrated Services Digital Network), which is OSI compliant and conforms with OSI layer 2 requirements. ISDN networks can carry all forms of communication: they use digital data streams and therefore permit connection of all manner of digital devices through an appropriate interface. Phones connected to ISDN must convert the analogue voice signal into digital form to send across the system. ISDN connections offer up to 30 data channels each of 64KBit capacity (plus one or two control channels), multiplexed and transmitted across wide-bandwidth media (e.g. optical fibres and microwave links).

Facsimile

Fax machines transmit a picture of a piece of paper rather like a photocopier where the original is one place but the copy emerges in quite another. They scan a "picture", strip by strip, to create a bit map of the page: each digitised strip of the picture is transformed into a format that is agreed for fax machine communications. When the machines first connect there is a "handshake" which establishes the communications protocol, following which data is sent, and the receiver acknowledges receipt or sends error messages. Because each page contains such a large amount of data when scanned in this way, the data is "compressed" before sending according to an algorithm: the algorithm is defined as another standard of CCITT. There are various algorithms for compression, some compressing the data more than others, and therefore sending the page faster: these are classified by "group" where the lower numbers (group 2) apply less data compression than higher numbers (group 3, group 4).

Other communications environments

OSI is not yet widely implemented, even though the potential for increased functionality and reduced interfacing costs are enormous. However, there is an entire collection of communications environments and technologies that are a legacy from the development of this area. At the most simple level, there are communications modalities that have little or no built-in reliability monitoring: these include some of the well known point-to-point MODEM links that you may have on your PC (as well as RS232 connections using V.24/V.28 protocols).

Two of the better known of the non-OSI communications protocols are Novell and TCP/IP (Transport Control Program/Internet Protocol), but almost every proprietary communicating or networked environment operates under its own specific communications protocol (e.g. IBM's SNA, SUN's NFS etc.). Each protocol of this type has its strengths and weaknesses: for example Novell is very functional on a local area, but is less suitable for wide area communications purposes.

At this point let us pursue the issue of the messages themselves, their syntax and general form.

Electronic messages

Housekeeping

Electronic messages must be highly structured if communications are to be effective. As an example, one might just be sending an item of electronic mail to a friend. If the message is to reach its destination, there must be an address that is in a predetermined position in the message (equivalent to addressing an envelope on the same side as the stamp), with the recipient's name first and the county/province, country and postcode last). The sender and origin address must also be identified so that an acknowledgment and reply can be sent.

The type of the message must be specified so that the receiving system knows how that message is structured and therefore how to read and interpret it (see below for message structure details).

The length of the message may also need to be specified so that intermediate stations handling it know that they must prepare and sequentially number an appropriate number of fixed-size packets, and the system knows when the communication is finished and the link can be broken. To mark the start and finish of each data element, and to distinguish it from the adjacent elements, a character is defined that will act as a **delimiter** and will be inserted between adjacent fields. Other special characters may be defined for specific purposes, such as to mark the end of a segment and/or of the entire message (**terminator**).

Each of these parameters must be sent with the message and placed in a predetermined location so that the systems know where to look for this important information. These data are usually placed in the message **header,** which precedes the content of the message.

Content and format

Consider an electronic bill sent to a purchaser of care services as a claim for care provided to a patient. As well as having the above information (sender and recipient names, address and NUA) for the purposes of ensuring that the message is delivered and acknowledged, the message must contain such data items as:

- the patient identification
- the items for which payment is claimed
- the date(s) when and place(s) where these services were rendered
- the amount of payment claimed
- the identity of the account to which payment is to be made

In order to make it possible to process such claims quickly and efficiently, the contents need to be laid out in a standard format, so that the receiving system can automatically scrutinise the message, detect errors and improbabilities, verify details (such as that the patient is insured by that purchaser, and the current reimbursement rates for those services), and dispatch funds to the correct account.

It is even necessary for the structure of the data within each of those defined data elements to conform to a pattern, so that, for example, the date might be required in the form "ccyymmdd" (e.g. 19930910 for the 10th September 1993), and the professional services rendered might be required in Read codes.

Take another example — the message from the laboratory providing the results of a request for a full blood count. This would also require a predetermined data set, laid out in a standard form. As well as the above details, the numeric values for the various types of blood cell, together with a text report would be included in the message. Say the haematocrit of the patient was 40 per cent: the figure '40' is therefore incorporated into the message. It is vital that the recipient should recognise this as a haematocrit value, and should not be able to mistake it for the platelet count ($\times 10,000$) or the patient age, or indeed any other element at all.

Any material that is not essential to the transmission is omitted, and the remaining content is reduced wherever possible to compact and concise codes. Using the same example of a full blood count message, the names of the attributes (e.g. "Total White Cell Count millilitre", or "Haemoglobin in grams per Litre") are predefined and therefore known to both sender and receiver: they are therefore not required to be transmitted. What is required is the value of that attribute in the full blood count.

Thus the following statements can be made about a message:

- every type of message has a defined purpose
- each message type requires a predefined set of data elements to fulfill that purpose
- every element has a defined meaning (e.g. in a national data dictionary)
- the data elements must be in a predefined position in the message, indicating to what they relate
- each data element must be presented in a predefined way (preferred format), and with predefined 'dimensions' (e.g. $\times 10,000$ cells per mm^3, grams/litre etc.)
- messages are kept as short as possible for four reasons:
  1. to minimise network traffic and therefore peak traffic capacity required
  2. to minimise connection times and therefore user costs
  3. to minimise the probability of an error arising in the transmission
  4. to make it easier to find an error in a rejected message.

Electronic Data Interchange (EDI) for health

Electronic data interchange is the process of automated exchange of messages for a specified purpose. The major uses of **EDI** have been for **A**dministration, **C**ommerce and **T**ransport, and hence the syntax, dictionary of elements, messages and message segments that constitute EDIFACT. However, the general EDI framework is applicable to any data sets and "business", and it seems pointless to reinvent wheels purely for medical data exchange purposes. Use of EDI standards can achieve error free, almost instantaneous exchange of data, without repetition of effort or waste of time, and at a significant cost saving.

Clearly it makes sense that there should be a set of defined standard message types for use over a health data network. These should be structured such that they each include every element that is required for that message. Some messages might be highly structured as outlined above, whilst others might have a block of "free text" as their major data element, for example a referral letter or a note to a colleague.

UN/EDIFACT

EDIFACT comprises a set of syntax rules (structure of messages) for construction of a message ready for sending, and a complete range of ready-to-use standard electronic messages. The segments of each message, the data elements of each segment, and the coding system for each data element are defined in the directory. In other words EDIFACT provides a wealth of infrastructure in the form of standard data elements (e.g. "first name"), composite data elements (e.g. "name and address"), and complete message segments (e.g. "personal identification segment"). These can then be "mixed and matched" in order to construct new messages quickly and easily.

An administrative process follows whereby a new message is notified to the EDIFACT Board, registered, notified to users world-wide, and so on.

EDIFACT is at present limited to use in "batch" mode: all the receiver can do automatically is to acknowledge receipt or send an error message. EDIFACT cannot (yet) support messaging where there is a need for full interactivity between two computer systems, for example searching a remote database for records matching a set of criteria.

Much of the need for health messaging can be satisfied with batch communications. However, within an institution where PAS, ADT, departmental, finance and laboratory systems need to communicate, there is often a need for interactivity.

Health Level Seven (HL7)

Interactive exchange of information can be achieved using HL7. The name is derived from the uppermost OSI application layer, which is numbered 7 in the OSI stack. HL7 has gained some acceptance, especially in North America, for passing information between host systems in the same environment, for example between the laboratory system, patient master index system and the financial management system.

The concepts of all messaging environments are broadly similar, although at the detailed level the rules for message construction, the data dictionaries and the syntax used may differ.

Message specification

A message is specified in terms of the variables or required **data elements,** and their length.

Consider a message segment for a full blood count report which has been defined, for this book, using the tilde (~) character as a field delimiter, the vertical bar (|) character as the segment terminator, and as having the following numeric field elements in this order (material in parentheses () define the format and dimensions for that element):

~DATE(ccyymmdd)~WBC(*10^5/ml)~RBC(*10^8/ml)~Hb(gm/dl)~HCT(%)
~MCV(*10^{-6})~MCH(pg/cell)~MCHC(gm/dl)~PLATELETS(*10^3/ml)
~E-PHILS~B-PHILS~MONO~LYMPHO~|

The actual message transmitted and received might be as follows:

~19930522~48~50~16~45~85~30~31~140~2~0~3~:20~|

If a data element is to be omitted from this "standard" message definition, the receiving station needs to be advised so that the variables which follow are placed in the right slots. For example, if the HCT were not measured for some reason, the message would be modified as below:

~220592~48~50~16~~~85~30~31~140~2~0~3~20~|

If another laboratory were to omit the entire differential white blood cell count (E-PHILS to the end), the message would be truncated with the segment terminator, as follows:

~220592~48~50~16~45~85~30~31~140~|

The message specification has to be agreed in common by both sender and receiver in order for the message to be communicated meaningfully. If, for example, laboratory 1 uses the above syntax, but laboratory 2 chooses to relocate the WBC figure between that for the PLATELETS and the E-PHILS, and to omit the MCHC figure, there is potential for confusion. That is why the message header must identify the type, version and source of the message being sent.

Elements are grouped together into **segments** for convenience: each segment contains elements that relate to one aspect of the message (e.g. patient identification). The advantage of building messages segmentally is that whole segments can be reused in other messages to avoid replication of effort, and to make new message creation quicker.

Within a message, each segment or element may be Mandatory (has to be present), Conditional (must be present when certain criteria are fulfilled) or Optional (need not be included). Each segment or element may appear only once, or may be repeated up to any number of times (e.g. the "diagnosis" element may need to be repeated up to 10 times to accommodate all relevant diagnoses for a patient).

Codes in messages

In all sorts of situations it is preferable to use codes to represent meanings, rather than to enter long "strings" of text. The reasons for this are simple:

- codes are concise and compact
- codes eliminate ambiguity
- codes are easily handled and "understood" by computers
- codes limit the infinity of possible entries that could be made
- codes force decisions and impose structure
- codes reduce the probability of errors
- codes make it possible to combine and compare data from different sources

Electronic messaging environments maintain large numbers of coding tables, and health is no exception to this. Not only will diagnoses be coded, but also a wide range of other attributes, such as occupation, ethnicity, domicile, medications, allergies and so on.

One code may often look very much like another — who is to know whether the code 31005 derives from coding system 1, where it might mean "diagnosis of acute myocardial infarction" or from coding system 2, where it could mean "ambulance transport required to home". Hence it is normal practice to qualify a code with a second code that identifies the coding system (date, version, release, original language etc.) used in the first code. Every code is presented as a couplet of "code" plus "coding system identifier": in some systems there may even be a third qualifying code to identify the organisation responsible for the maintenance of that coding system (e.g. WHO in the case of ICD9).

Validation of messages

Sending messages around a network that are meaningless would be wasteful and would generate an equal number of error messages from the recipient systems: far better to check the message before sending for validity. Each element in a message normally has a defined set of valid values: other values are not acceptable in the context of that specific message. The message construction tools are normally designed to check the valid values or coding tables for each element before preparing a message for sending.

Chapter 11 Security and privacy

Data is the most valuable asset of the health sector after the staff themselves. The protection of these data from loss or damage, and ensuring their availability to those who need access to them, is vital to the management of the business and to the care of patients at all levels. This chapter is longer than many others in this book, reflecting the high priority that the authors place on this issue. It is not an issue that can ever be left to "someone else": everyone must be aware of the issues. The security of your system is no better than that of its weakest part.

Communications and linkages of various sorts between computers are set to become an increasingly important part of the routine delivery of health care. Sharing of data and resources must always be based upon trust. You must be able to trust anyone with whom you share private and confidential data to respect it as you would wish them to, and vice versa. You must be able to trust anyone who makes use of your computer system to behave in the way you intended when you authorised that level of access and as a user of a system you must respect the trust placed in you by the owners of that system and of the data stored in it, and not abuse their trust in you.

What is security?

The need for security arises out of risks or threats. Like with insurance, when everything is going well there seems to be no need for security: it is only when disaster strikes that the absence of security measures is really appreciated. Security is a set of preventive measures and proactive steps taken to guard against risks and preserve:

- system **integrity** — the functionality of the computer system should be maintained with all modules and subsystems functioning properly and in the way that user expects and believes them to be operating
- data **availability** — the data stored is preserved from damage or disorganisation, and is available to the user as and when he/she requires

- information **privacy** — the personal and confidential material stored is protected from access by unauthorised personnel, and is available only to those with a need to know and with the necessary privilege and authority to access it

All computers are at risk to a greater or lesser extent. At some point in their life every computer will experience a malfunction, and in many instances this generates a significant potential for data to be lost or damaged. The amount of resources expended on security systems will depend upon

- their perceived vulnerability or exposure to risk
- their perceived importance and value to their users

Computer systems are now essential to the day-to-day operation of most companies. Indeed, it has been claimed that 70 per cent of all UK companies would have to cease trading if they lost their computers for more than two days[1], and some businesses such as those providing telephone banking and credit vetting would have to stop immediately if their computers were down. However, in too many instances it is not until disaster has struck that the real value of the systems and their data, and the impact of their non-availability, is recognised, but by then it is too late.

Why is security so important?

Security has always been an important issue since records started being kept. Considerable effort is devoted to securing premises where records are stored in paper folders, and to ensuring that only those personnel who are authorised have access to the files. There is normally only one copy of a paper record, and it is stored in a specific location: the risk of a breach of security passing undetected can be made relatively low by ensuring physical oversight of records and of those with access to them.

Unauthorised amendments can be made to paper records, but methods exist for their detection (e.g. analyses of paper, ink, handwriting etc.). However, in spite of this it has proven relatively easy for individuals to access records without authorisation in the past, and, frequently, to take the records away with them for copying. Every records department can give numerous examples of such incidents, and those are just the instances that have been detected.

Electronic records, however, can easily be read, copied and amended from a remote location: indeed this is one of their advantages, but it is also a potential problem. The user is normally unseen, the file access may pass unnoticed, and any changes that are made may well remain undetected. The growing numbers of individuals

---

[1] Source: Price Waterhouse Disaster Planning and Recovery Seminar, 1991

who possess the necessary familiarity with computer systems to be able to carry out these hostile attacks with the minimum of investment in technology serves only to exacerbate the threat.

The risk of unauthorised access is considerable, and therefore there needs to be concomitantly greater investment in system security. However, the benefits of secure storage of records in electronic formats are considerable, since it becomes much easier to find them, sort them, analyse them, communicate them to other professionals and so on, and because the manual tasks of checking the records in and out, and chasing them when they are lost, are eliminated.

Security risks

The common risks which security systems and procedures must protect against are:

- physical attack, for example fire, theft or flood, unavailability of systems, for example power or component failure, virus attack or software crash
- loss of confidentiality, unauthorised disclosure of information

In many instances the consequences of a breach of security will be self-evident. However, it is increasingly common for security to be breached without the owner or operator of the system being aware of it. Data may be read by unauthorised personnel and files may be copied, deleted or modified without the security breach being detected.

This highlights the benefit of two key features of security systems. One is the ability to keep a log of all transactions so that it is possible to "roll-back" to any point in the past and follow the transactions that took place one by one. The other is to identify and keep track of users in order to limit their access and to keep a record of what they do. These may be more important to larger systems with many users, but the issues are still just as relevant to systems of all sizes.

Consequences of breach of security

The consequences are the same regardless of whether the records are on paper or in electronic form, and whether the system is small or large. Where the breach is significant, the loss that results may be measurable in financial terms, but may also have components that are less readily quantifiable, but no less important, such as:

- harm to personal health and safety
- personal and corporate embarrassment and loss of goodwill
- infringement of personal privacy
- failure to meet obligations, especially legal and contractual obligations
- loss of commercial confidentiality and commercially sensitive data
- disruption to normal business operations

Some of the typical consequences that may arise from lapses of security are:

- decisions about patient care may be delayed or inappropriate, and the consequences for the patient could be very serious if records are lost, inaccessible or altered. Simple failure of the Patient Administration System, for example, may make it virtually impossible to locate the record for an individual
- calculations performed by computer, for example of drug or radiation dosages, may be erroneous if the computer is not available, or the software is malfunctioning: the possible consequences for the patient and therefore for the provider are serious
- litigation for breach of personal privacy and for any damage suffered as a consequence may be expected where personal information is accessed by unauthorised individuals, or it is disclosed improperly
- clinics may have to be cancelled where patient records cannot be located
- it may not be possible to process staff pay, or draw up rosters
- communications may be paralysed if the computer or software operating the exchange malfunctions, and disasters may result
- loss of clinical or financial records may drive a unit into receivership

Up-to-date information and knowledge are the most important assets available to the provider of care services. It is vital to ensure that these resources are securely protected, and that they are available and functioning properly whenever they are required.

Security policy

At the uppermost level, a security policy is required which should cover all of the precautions which each organisation needs to follow to ensure integrity, availability and confidentiality of its information assets. This is a business issue rather than a strictly technical problem. The responsibility for planning and implementation of appropriate security measures lies with management, and it is a responsibility of top management to ensure that these responsibilities are taken seriously at every level of an organisation.

The value of the information environment to the users is potentially very high: their reliance on computerised systems to provide information upon demand will increase. Computers are becoming indispensable in the highly information-intensive business of delivering high quality health care services and managing an efficient business. But for this to happen the computer systems must be perceived as secure, trustworthy and reliable.

The risk of essential data loss or system failure is an issue which, for reasons that will become clear, cannot be addressed in a piecemeal way since systems are more and more interdependent. There must be a coherent approach to ensure that all threats and risks are identified, evaluated and effectively managed.

Security principles

In recent years various philosophical and functional approaches to systems security issues have been formulated, and these have been drawn together by the OECD as a series of statements of principle. Amongst these are the following:

- **awareness** — to foster confidence in their information systems, all users should be knowledgeable and informed about security practices and procedures
- **accountability** — the responsibilities and accountability of owners, providers and users of information systems should be explicit with regard to security
- **proportionality** — security levels and countermeasures should be appropriate and proportionate to the value of and degree of reliance upon those systems, and to the severity, probability and extent of potential harm that might result from breach of security
- **reassessment** — security should be reassessed at frequent intervals as systems are modified, technology evolves and risks and potential consequences of security breaches alter
- **democracy** — system security and data accessibility should be compatible with the legitimate needs for and flow of data and information in an open and democratic society
- **integration** — there should be coherent and integrated approaches to security throughout all elements of an information system
- **timeliness** — all parties should co-operate with each other to prevent and respond quickly to breaches of security, especially where the breach may involve a user on another system

These principles are self-explanatory. It would clearly be inappropriate to secure information to the extent that legitimate users were unable to gain access to the information as and when they had need of it. It would be ill-advised to link computers together into networks if everyone expects someone else to sort out security for the system, or if some nodes of the network make no effort to secure their systems, thus putting the security of the entire network at risk. There must be a general agreement about what is appropriate in terms of security and who is responsible for implementation of what counter-measures. This is especially important where networks link together different jurisdictions: cooperation agreements between systems managers must ensure that offenders can be identified and apprehended despite their belonging to different organisations and perhaps to different countries.

System availability and integrity

Maintaining system availability and functionality is a major issue. A system that continually lets you down when you most need it is of little value and is not trusted by its users with important information. Where users do not trust a system, they end up keeping parallel files on paper in order to maintain a degree of independence, and so that there is at least something to work from when the system fails next time. Often the paper files are kept more up to date than the computer, further reducing its usefulness.

Systems become unavailable because, for example:

- the power supply fails
- an internal system hardware component fails
- an external component or interface to another system (e.g. telecommunications link) fails
- the software "hangs", probably due to a "bug", a software interaction or a virus
- new software is installed before it has been subjected to sufficiently rigorous testing
- the system becomes overloaded with major computational tasks
- the operations manager chooses to carry out maintenance or a back-up at peak use time

Simple remedies to maintain system availability are:

- install an uninterruptible power supply (a battery power unit for when the mains supply fails)
- implement a service and maintenance agreement which guarantees hardware repairs within a defined time period
- implement a service agreement with the software vendor or agent which includes hot line support, regular software updates and guarantees of functionality for your software
- ensure that there is a very recent back-up of the software so that if a memory device is destroyed, it can quickly be installed and reconfigured like the old one
- plan routine system housekeeping for times when transactions are at a minimum (e.g. weekends, overnight)
- ensure major processing tasks are restricted to low usage times
- ensure adequate processor capacity for peak user loads and periods through appropriate planning

More complex remedies include, for example:

- RAID disk configurations, where failure of any one disk in a multi-disk array causes no loss of functionality of data (see below)
- complete duplication of systems, with one operating and the other acting as a "hot" back-up site ready to take over at a moment's notice.

RAID stands for Redundant Array of Inexpensive Disks and is classified in five levels. At the simplest level a "mirrored" disk assembly can be used. In this arrangement data is written first to one disk, and then milliseconds later to the other. Each disk has an exact copy of the data on the other, so that if one fails the other can take over without loss of function. In its most complex form, RAID systems can spread the data across a number of disks, in such a way that the data lost through failure of any one disk can be reconstituted from the remaining data and check data.

Data integrity

In more complex computing environments there may be a risk of muddles arising between systems. Where a database (e.g. of patient names, addresses and record numbers) is used by many people, there are often multiple local copies of sub-sets of that database held in different places, since it is often easier and faster to access, process and modify a local database than a remote one. As data is added or amended, it is vital for the systems to know which database is the "master" or primary store, and which are just copies or secondary stores. The significance of the master database is that it must receive all updated information from all clients: it can then take steps to broadcast updates to all secondary stores. Where this does not happen, the databases will soon diverge and data integrity in the environment will be lost: in other words different systems "know" different details about the same individual. People using different systems in the same location will be provided different, and often conflicting, information about the subject.

Confidentiality

System confidentiality is absolutely essential in healthcare. If there is any suspicion that data is not treated as confidential, people will either refuse to provide information, will adopt aliases, or will deliberately supply erroneous, incomplete or misleading information. As the data quality starts to fall, so the value and utility of the system plummets also.

The issue of privacy as a whole is addressed in detail below.

Security counter-measures

Access control

The simplest approach to systems access control is **physical security:** where the system and all its components can be kept behind locked doors the risk of unauthorised use is small. However, tight physical security often adversely impacts on the principle of democracy and the need for system availability and flexibility. The location of terminals should be reviewed in the light of their physical security, for example by placement where the user can be visually monitored. The screen should be placed such that the user can easily read the display, but it is hidden from others.

Physical access to the system servers and operations console should be restricted by appropriate physical measures (e.g. locks), and steps taken to ensure that any network components (wiring trunks, outlets) are also secured (e.g. underground, in locked cupboards etc.). Software, back-ups, configuration information, source code, security information and password files should be physically secured also, normally in a fireproof safe. However, there is a limit to what can reasonably be done to improve physical security without it impinging significantly on flexibility and utility.

149

A key feature of almost every system, large or small, is some form of **system log in** process, followed by authentication (e.g. a password). Users are normally required to negotiate access rights with the owner of the computer system, or set up an "account" or "userID". This negotiation determines just what they are permitted to do and use within the system (and often also determines a scale of charges). Operations staff can then establish a table of access rights for each user, which means that whenever that user then logs into the system, the files he/she can read, write (i.e. update, modify and delete) and execute (i.e. software applications) are pre-set.

Passwords, tokens and PINs

The key to access comes at the time of login, when the authorised user has to identify him/herself to the system. The elements of this identification process comprise up to three parts:

- something you know (e.g. a password)
- something you have (e.g. a token)
- something unique to you (e.g. a fingerprint)

Many systems use just the first of these (e.g. a password associated with userID), which may be adequate with proper management. But unless passwords are changed frequently, are kept secret and are difficult to guess they are useless.

In many institutions several users may share the same account and password: in other situations one user may be able to quote the user names and passwords of several different individuals. Other institutions may have userIDs which relate to a function (e.g. MEDREG for duty medical registrar), with little idea as to who the user at any specific time may be. Examples of such practices abound in the health sector. The authors are aware of one institution where all medical staff share the same userID and password, neither of which have been changed for almost a decade. Other user names and passwords are so obvious that anyone could guess them (e.g. password same as username, password is own firstname, password for lab tests is LAB or HAEM or PATH etc.). Unless you can be certain who is the user at any specific point in time, every attempt to enforce ethical and behavioural standards (see below) must fail.

A typical suite of passwords might provide the following access to a specific application for different classes of system user:

1. system Manager and Operations staff — all functions
2. systems Programmer or Developer — all functions except control of user access and deletion of any data
3. editor — read and write other's records
4. researcher, quality assurance — read only other's records

5. author — edit own records
6. data entry clerk — write only
7. others — no access

This highlights a specific problem in that information services staff (systems manager, operations staff, programmers etc.) have wide powers of access to data and programs, which may prove an irresistible temptation and may require special provisions for supervision, audit and shared responsibilities.

Most systems have the capacity to impose a "timeout" function whereby a terminal is disconnected if no keys have been pressed for a preset time interval. Some may also enforce the abrupt termination of a session connection if three attempts to log in or provide a valid password have been unsuccessful.

Access to networks and shared facilities/files

When a computer is linked in to a network, as will be the case in almost every installation in the near future, the resources of that computer are vulnerable to attack from remote locations as well as from the local terminals. This highlights the need for conjoint approaches to security, involving both your system and any other system that is able to link in and make use of its resources. The nature of the links to be established with other systems needs careful consideration to ensure that there is adequate provision for transaction logging and audit trails (see below), and that the approaches to security used by third-party systems are consistent with your own. There is a need to reach agreements so that there is a degree of mutual comfort between the owners of the systems that are networked. Practices for exchanging information in order to identify abusers must be set in place.

Hackers

A determined hacker can employ technology that will eventually, by the laws of probability, break in to most systems which are secured only by characters entered on a keyboard. There is now much interest and various pilot studies on the use of physical tokens, or "keys", such as "smart" cards for additional security coupled with ease of access for the authorised user.

Various techniques such as disconnection of a terminal for a period of time after three consecutive access attempts have failed is sometimes adopted, but impacts on the utility of terminals and only delays the determined hacker. Careful surveillance for abnormal and exceptional patterns of activity is probably the best way to detect hackers, as well as to identify authorised users who appear to be making unusual and suspicious transactions.

Transaction logs and audit trails

Once a user has been positively identified it becomes possible to implement either of two philosophical strategies for prevention of abuse of privilege: preventive or detective. The preventive strategy aims to limit the capacity for abuse by identifying categorically what the user can and cannot do, and rigidly enforcing these restrictions. The detective strategy recognises that often users may have a need to do things that had not been anticipated, and so aims to permit greater flexibility and user discretion. However, every transaction is tracked and logged. This log file can be subject to routine surveillance of activity patterns, as well as to detailed study where an abuse is alleged or suspected. Detection can be assured.

Every sensitive or important file should have an audit trail of changes made. For every entry or alteration in that file, the trail should indicate at the very least who authorised the transaction and when. In terms of the requirements for evidence that could be used in a court of law, audit trails are invaluable.

Encryption

Links between computers, for example telephone lines, radio, micro-wave and satellite links, are vulnerable to attack and interception. Data sent by conventional mail is also at risk, and should always be consigned to secure services for delivery. Where the data is sensitive, it may be wise to "scramble" or encrypt it in some way, as the military have been doing for centuries. It may not be necessary to scramble the entire message: encryption of just those items which identify the individual may be enough.

The process of encryption may be carried out in many ways, for example by adding or subtracting a fixed or a variable number from the (digital value of the) character to be encrypted.

This renders the data meaningless to anyone who does not know the "key". On arrival at the destination the receiver decrypts the message using the same key (symmetrical or single key encryption) or a complementary but different key (asymmetrical or dual key encryption). Where a large number of computers are involved, a single key ends up so widely distributed that almost anyone can get access to it, so its security value is lost. For this reason asymmetrical encryption is the safest and most secure. Management of asymmetrical encryption is an exercise in the secure management of the keys. Each user is assigned two keys: a **private** key which the user keeps secret, and a **public** key which is widely distributed, for example in directories of users. Data encrypted with either of the keys can only be decrypted with the other key. The obvious choice for management of these keys is to keep them in a secure device, such as a smart card: any number of secret keys or PINs can be held in such a device, secured by the single user password to the smart card (for further material on smart cards, see also discussion of PHMR devices in chapter 8).

Dual key encryption works because although the private and public keys are mathematically related to each other, any attempt to determine the value of one from the other is for all practical purposes impossible. Whilst in principle any encryption algorithm can be broken, in practice even a very simple algorithm presents a difficult, complex and costly cryptographic task that few would be able or willing to undertake. Two approaches to encryption algorithms may be adopted: use of a publicly known routine which has the benefit of extensive testing; or use of a locally developed routine, which may not be well tested but has the advantage of being completely unknown. A public standard for encryption, called DES — Data Encryption Standard — is well tried and tested and resists most attempts at deciphering.

The processes of encryption and decryption impose a processing overhead and therefore increase costs and times.

The three main applications of encryption are:

- **encrypted messages** — message encryption is quite straightforward. The sender encrypts each message with the public key of the recipient. The recipient decrypts the message using his/her private key

- **electronic signature** — electronic signatures provide a guarantee as to the originator of a document. When a user signs a document, his/her ID number is encrypted using the **private** key. The receiver decrypts this field using the public key of that user. If the IDs match, the signature is verified and could only have been affixed by that individual. This process can be applied to any materials, for example notes entries in electronic medical records, orders and so on — anywhere that the identity of the originator must be confirmed

- **protection of sensitive data** — sensitive data can be encrypted in such a way that only a specified set of individuals can obtain access to it. In this situation, the encryption is specified by the database designer, and all users who need access to this data require an encryption key. It is quite possible for any one user to have a number of special encryption keys, each permitting access to a different class of data or a different group of user files.

Archiving

Part of the issue of data protection relates to the ease with which it is accessible. All data that is not currently required, or does not need to be instantly accessible can be readily protected by "off-line" storage, that is by archiving to a device (disk or tape) that has to be physically loaded onto a computer before it can be read.

Data archives must be stored securely, for example in a fireproof safe (see under back-ups).

Destruction

Where personal data has fulfilled its purposes, it should be destroyed as required by privacy principles. Paper records should be shredded on site to eliminate the possibility of accidental breach of confidence. Data stored on electronic devices, for example hard or floppy disks, must be erased. Simple "delete" commands are not sufficient, since the file can normally be recovered with appropriate utilities: the device must be reformatted to ensure that all traces of the data are destroyed.

Systems engineering

Where computer systems or memory devices require maintenance or repair, all the data stored on them is placed at risk of disclosure to the service personnel. This process must be monitored and supervised closely. Inserting a non-disclosure clause into the service contract is unlikely to achieve anything but a sense of false security: it is more important to prevent such a breach.

Software Issues: virus protection and software fitness

It is possible for those with appropriate skills and experience to develop and modify software to function in ways that are potentially undesirable and/or not immediately obvious. One example is the introduction of various types of destructive computer code, such as "viruses". It is becoming easier for those with minimal expertise to acquire software for automated virus development, and opportunities for their accidental or deliberate introduction into a system are many. Countermeasures in the form of central virus detection utilities can be adopted to counter this threat, but virus development will continue to lead detective measures by a significant margin.

As software is more widely used in support of patient care decisions and planning processes, it becomes increasingly important to ensure that the software is appropriate for those purposes, especially in critical environments. Some process of certification of software is required to confirm its suitability for the intended purpose and quality assurance to check for hidden bugs or unexpected outcomes should be implemented. This is particularly important where software has been developed or modified in-house, and especially in relation to the burgeoning quantities of microcomputer software.

Software is continuously being modified on large systems by information services personnel. It is possible for them to implement routines which modify applications in inappropriate ways and which may pass undetected. It is important to ensure that modifications are checked by a supervisor. Adequate documentation of all changes must be made for audit requirements, as an integral element of quality management processes, and for the future operational management of the system and software.

Back-ups

The simplest of precautions that every user of a computer should use is that of making a back-up copy of programs and data. If there is a system failure, the last complete back-up, together with any more recent selective back-ups will restore the system, excepting the transactions made since that back-up was made.

Backing up is the process of writing all the material on your computer to an off-line device, such as floppy disks or a tape drive. They could be written to an optical device for maximum durability. A complete back-up copies all data: for a system storing large amounts of data this may be a slow process and result in long periods of system unavailability. Even if scheduled for periods of low computer usage this still presents an availability problem. However, a back-up can be selective, simply copying all material that has been changed since the date of the last back-up. Many operating systems set an "archive" bit in the file attributes table when a file has been changed, and reset it when that file has been backed-up. Back-up security routines must be followed with obsessive zeal. All data held on disks should be backed up onto tape cartridges for safekeeping. There are two types of cartridge now available known as **QIC** (quarter inch cartridge) and **DAT** (Digital Audio Tape). QIC has capacity up to 500 Mb, while DAT can store over 2 Gb on a cartridge little bigger than a match box.

Backups are a protection against hardware or software problems which can have catastrophic results. Such disasters are rare, but it is essential to maintain more than one copy of all data and programs, and to ensure that making security copies is part of the daily routine. The frequency of back-up is determined by the maximum amount of data you are willing to lose, and the importance that you place on having all data and transactions available for medico-legal purposes.

A fire-proof safe should be used for storage of important information and back-up media (see below): this acts as a protection against both fire and water damage. The safe should include recent data backups and master copies of software including all application programs and the operating system. The fire-proof safe should also be used to keep safely all activation keys and special passwords needed to set up the system. It is often advisable to keep a copy of important materials off site for added protection.

Microcomputer security

There is no fundamental difference between a large computer and a small one, between a mainframe and a PC notebook in terms of their capability to store and access information and to be the vehicle whereby security infringements occur. Logically and legally they are the same. The only observable differences are that microcomputers often proliferate in a seemingly uncontrolled way, are operated and programmed by users whose awareness of security and quality assurance issues is minimal and frequently seem to be viewed as independent information empires even when linked in to extensive computer networks.

The fact that microcomputers are cheap, common, small and easy to use by those without any background in information technology must not be allowed to obscure the potential threat they may pose to data protection, personal privacy and system security. Some of the more widely used microcomputer operating systems designed for stand-alone usage may not be well suited to management of system security issues, although the development of multi-user and local area networking software has in many instances addressed this problem.

Security and people

Fundamental to any attempt to secure an information system is that the users are aware of and follow appropriate routines and prescribed procedures. It will remain beyond the realms of practical reality to develop preventive strategies that make it impossible for an authorised user to breach security, and it is the authorised users of the system who are the weakest link in the security system.

User policy

All organisations should have fully developed top level security policies. These should address the vulnerabilities and risks to security and identify individual responsibilities in supporting and maintaining security. They should also identify how abusers of the system will be identified and what steps will be taken to discipline offenders. Essential to any security policy is the development of strategies for the education of users. Obviously the need for and detail in such policies decreases where the organisation is small or single handed, although even small practices should pay careful attention to security issues.

User education and awareness

Clear rules and regulations for the security of any system, large or small, must be developed. The system manager must be satisfied that users are aware of the issues and the countermeasures, and periodic audits must be implemented to check on compliance. This is probably the most fundamental element of the entire security system.

Management responsibilities

The responsibility for planning and implementing appropriate security measures must lie with management. Specific responsibilities of managers include:

- placing emphasis on security and so creating a workplace that is aware and conscious of security and potential risks to security, and of the value of information
- development of a security policy
- ensuring that all individuals who make use of the information resources are fully aware of their responsibilities and follow the guidelines in the security policy
- implementing a security monitoring project, with the appointment (in larger organisations) of security officers, and the implementation of transaction logs and audit trails where software considerations permit

Management must also take responsibility for ensuring the compliance of those who are best placed to abuse security — the staff programming, servicing and operating the computer system. They have the opportunity, the access rights, the knowledge and the skills to create havoc, and, in many cases, to cover their tracks or shift the blame onto others.

The broad outline of steps that should be considered in the development of a security policy are outlined below:

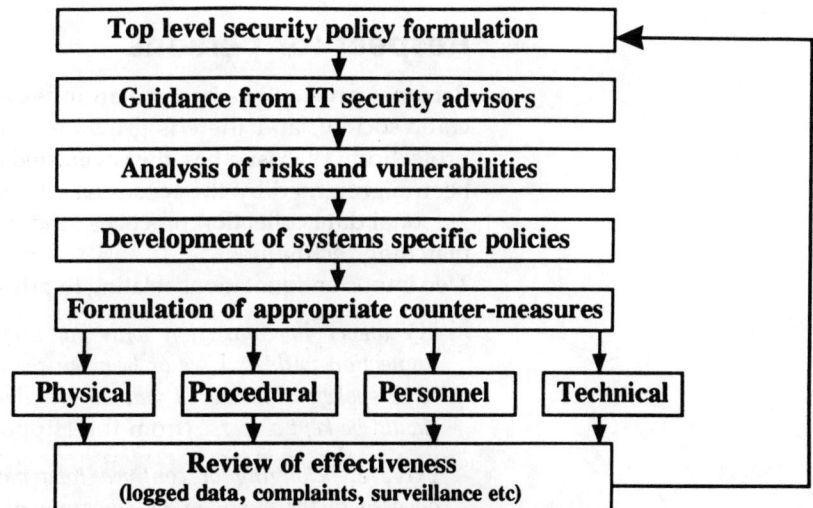

Figure 11.1 Development of a security policy

Privacy

Illnesses and other health events are by their very nature an extremely private matter for an individual, going to the very heart of personal space, self-esteem and identity. It is essential and inevitable that health professionals must, sensitively but purposefully, invade to some extent that privacy in order to make accurate diagnoses and plan appropriate care. This is the essence of medical practice, and is understood by both parties to a care encounter. The increasing complexity and scientific precision of medicine means that often more data is required than in the past to reach decisions, and that it may need to be shared between a larger team of professionals involved in the care of each individual.

There is rapid growth in the development and deployment of electronic information systems in hospitals and clinics of all types, a deployment that took place in many other sectors as long as 20 years ago. There is a wealth of experience from which to infer what is likely to happen and where the problems are likely to arise. This section addresses specificially the issues of privacy and confidentiality of personally identifying information. There is clear evidence of concern in the community over this issue.

If there is any suspicion that the privacy and confidentiality of personal information is not protected, the quantity and quality of the information provided willingly by individuals (patient and providers) will rapidly fall, and the value and benefits of the information system will be markedly reduced. This will lead to degradation in the integrity and continuity of care provided to individuals, as well as to less and poorer quality information for management. A datastore is only as good as the quality of the information within it, and thus the datastore itself becomes worthless. It is now widely accepted that making adequate provision for personal privacy protection in a datastore is a sound economic investment.

Respect for persons

Personal privacy has become an index of political freedom in democratic society, and there is growing concern about personal privacy protection. The issue has always existed and been recognised, but has been highlighted by the recent trend towards increasingly sweeping personal data collection practices, and greater use of data linking and matching techniques.

Two important quotations relating to privacy and confidentiality follow:

> "Whatever in connection with my professional practice, or not in connection with it, I see or hear, in the life of men, which ought not to be spoken of abroad, I will not divulge, as reckoning that all such should be kept secret." (from the Hippocratic Oath)

> **Private:** belonging or confined to a particular person or group as opposed to the public or the government; Known about by very few. (Dictionary Definition)

The basis of information privacy

There is a generally recognised right of individuals to three forms of privacy:

- privacy of person (from assault and violence)
- privacy of personal property (from theft and damage)
- privacy of personal information

Almost everyone resents intrusions into their personal privacy (even though they often seem to delight in intrusions into the privacy of others, for example by the popular media). A legitimate tension exists between the right of the individual to privacy and the right of the community and others to obtain information by whatever means.

Respect for personal information

It has long been accepted that the information that passes between two individuals in certain types of encounter is given and received for one specific purpose. It should remain private and not be disclosed to anyone else at all. Examples of this recognition relate to information passed to a priest in the confessional, communications between lawyer and client, the expectation that journalists will protect their sources of information, and, of course, the understanding that anything said to a doctor in the course of a professional encounter will remain a secret.

But can the individual rely on the person to whom he/she divulges information in connection with a health care encounter treating it with due respect? This is not just an issue for the patient: the provider may also have occasion to supply private and/or commercially sensitive information to purchasers, government and statutory authorities.

There is a general expectation that the individual has the right to control who knows what about him or her, with certain exceptions. There has always been some measure of legal protection for personal information privacy, but it has been patchy and disorganised, with gaping holes in places. Some communications have been designated as legally privileged (e.g. discussion between lawyer and client), but health care information has not been so protected. Some public sector employment contracts have required employees to respect confidences.

Where breach of privacy could be shown to have elements of bribery and corruption there has been a basis for legal redress. It has also been possible to lodge a complaint against an offending provider alleging unprofessional conduct. However, in most cases the subject of the breach has been powerless to seek any significant redress.

Privacy legislation is being enacted worldwide at the present time, reflecting the levels of concern over the issue. Despite this there are many specific legislative jurisdictions where personal information still remains incompletely protected.

Natural history of information

The natural history of information is best viewed in terms of the processes of:

- **gathering** — the collection of personal data from subjects and others
- **storage** — the aggregation and cataloguing of information for systematic retrieval in secure storage
- **maintenance** — keeping records of information stored, and keeping the stored information accurate, adequate for the purpose and up-to-date
- **access and use** — determination of who may access and use the information, and for what purposes
- **destruction** — rendering the information useless
- **disclosure** — determination of to whom information may be passed and under what circumstances

In 1981 the OECD drafted guidelines for the transborder flow of data based on a series of broad principles. These principles have been widely accepted internationally as the basis for personal privacy protection. A brief summary of the thrust of these internationally accepted guidelines follows.

1. **purpose of collection of personal information** — information may only be collected for a lawful purpose connected with a function or activity of the collecting agency, and must be necessary for that purpose to be fulfilled. This underlines the "need to know" principle, that it is essential to know this information in order to provide the care service
2. **source of health information** — information should normally be collected directly from the individual concerned, although there are a number of possible exemptions to this rule, including where the individual is not able to provide the necessary information (e.g. an infant, an unconscious person etc.). Where an exemption is invoked, the source from which the information is obtained must be recorded. This rule ensures that individuals have control over who knows what about them, and tries also to ensure its accuracy
3. **solicitation of information from the individual concerned** — the individual should be made aware before the event of the fact that the information is to be collected for storage, the purpose(s) of its collection, the intended use and recipients of the information, whether or not they are required to provide the information, and the consequences of not providing all or part of it. It is assumed that routine collection of information in order to provide care services to the patient requires no further explanation to the patient, but that any information collected for other purposes, or for disclosure to third parties, should be explicitly stated. There is no need to restate these details where a repeat encounter of an essentially similar type takes place

4. **solicitation of personal information generally** — information should not be collected by means that are unlawful, unfair or unreasonably intrusive into personal affairs. Whilst collection of very sensitive information may be necessary, it should be collected in physical privacy by appropriately briefed and culturally sensitive persons and without unnecessary repetition. Lawfulness of collection implies that it is collected in accordance with an appropriate authority or purpose, and fairness implies that all these principles are observed. The aim of this rule is to prevent undue pressure being applied to individuals to provide information

5. **storage and security of health information** — information must be stored with adequate protection against loss and unauthorised access, modification, disclosure or other misuse. This requirement to protect the information applies also where the information is made available to another person providing services to the same patient, and every precaution must be taken to ensure that that this does not result in compromise to its security. There are issues of physical, operational and technical systems security involved in compliance with this principle

6. **information relating to personal information kept by an agency** — agencies should maintain documentation as to the information that they hold, the persons or institutions who have access to that data and the conditions under which they can exercise that access, and the steps that should be taken by individuals wishing to obtain access to their own information

7. **access to own personal health information** — where information is held such that it can be readily retrieved, the subject must be able to find out that it is held and have access to it in order to check on its accuracy, with a right to request that corrections be made where appropriate (see 8 below). Access must be granted within a defined period, and generally no charges can be made for this access. There are various bases for refusing access

8. **correction of personal health information** — where an individual requests correction of his/her stored personal information, it should be corrected as long as that correction does not interfere with the purpose of collection: if the incorrect information has been disclosed to others, where practicable they should be advised of the correction sought and/or made. Where the correction is refused, a note must be attached in such a way as always to be read with the data itself indicating the correction requested but not made. Where the correction relates to an integral element of the medical record upon which clinical or administrative decisions may have been based, alteration to the record would be ill advised unless an adequate audit trail were in place to permit the original record to be retrieved for evidence and other purposes. The objective of this rule is to ensure that decisions are taken based on accurate information.

9. **access to reasons for decisions** — where a decision is taken based on personal information held, the individual concerned is entitled to an explanation of the reasons for that decision

10. **agency to check accuracy of personal information before use** — information held must be checked before it is used to ensure that it is accurate, up-to-date, complete, relevant and not misleading. This is so as to ensure that all decisions taken are based on full and current information

11. **agency not to keep information for longer than necessary** — information should be kept only for as long as it is still required for a legitimate use (see principle 12 for limits on use). Where it is no longer needed it must be disposed of in such a way as to make it irretrievable and unreadable. Clinical information may need to be retained for some time, and perhaps for life and even for some time after death: archiving of information that is being kept purely for medico-legal reasons in such a way that it is less readily accessible can contribute to reducing the burden that this information might present. Where a professional is leaving a practice, the records should still be retained and should be disposed of as far as possible in accord with the wishes of the patients concerned. They might be left with the patient, with another doctor of the patient's choice, or with the district Medical Officer of Health

12. **limits on the use of health information** — in essence this rule restricts the use of information collected to the use(s) that were disclosed as the reason for its collection (see principle 1), and for which the subject assented to its collection. There are a number of exceptions (see Code of Practice document, notably where the individual assents to its other use, or where the information is deemed necessary to prevent or lessen a serious and imminent threat to public health, public safety, or to the life and health of the individual concerned or of another individual

13. **limits on disclosure of health information** — essentially the same principles apply as in the previous rule. The information may not be disclosed unless its disclosure in this way was one of the declared purposes of its collection, or disclosure is to the individual concerned, or authorised by him/her, or as outlined under principle 12 above

Confidentiality of information in contracting

The development of contracting between purchasers and providers continues to generate many new uses for information. It is important to ensure that these new uses are supported, but not at the expense of loss of privacy protection. Information used to support contracting is confidential and must be subject to the same safeguards as any other information that identifies individuals directly or indirectly. Personalised information used in connection with contracting must be restricted to that which is essential for the purpose(s) and no more, and access to this information must be governed by the "need to know" principle.

Much of the information could and should be processed without the identity of the individuals being revealed: patients can be identified by numbers, encrypted where necessary, to protect their identity where it is not needed. Wherever possible the same person should not be in a position to know both clinical details and the identity of the individual to whom they relate.

Management and privacy

Privacy is a responsibility of top level management. In addition to the security measures outlined above, some of the steps in implementing an appropriate privacy management plan should include:

- developing an **institutional privacy policy** and publicising it
- taking steps to ensure that all **staff are fully briefed** on the provisions of privacy as they affect them, and on all relevant provisions of the institutional privacy policy
- reviewing all **standard forms** requesting information in the light of the principles
- reviewing standard **operating procedures** in every area of the institution in the context of Privacy
- carrying out a **stocktake of what personalised information** is held, why, and for how much longer it is required, ensuring that all microcomputer-based systems are included in this stocktake
- developing **procedures for routine culling and disposal** of unwanted records, preferably in the first instance by offering them to the subjects of the records
- developing procedures for furnishing individuals with **access to their own information,** and for acting upon requests for amendments to their records
- developing procedures for the **management of requests for disclosure** of information
- developing programs for **monitoring privacy compliance**
- **reviewing access to personal information** by all staff, including information services and computing staff
- establishment of **"dummy"** data resources for the purposes of staff training and testing of software
- identification of where **responsibility** lies for specific aspects of privacy compliance, including appointment of responsible security officers

Chapter 12   Education, audit and research

The practice of medicine is enormously information intensive. The successful practice of contemporary medicine requires not just that the care provider knows a vast amount of information, but that he/she can identify and access relevant items at random from this in the context of a specific patient problem, and has the expertise to apply them appropriately to that context.

The knowledge base of medicine is constantly expanding: what was accurate and adequate in terms of knowledge and understanding during undergraduate studies is often proven to be inaccurate and/or inadequate a few years later. As a profession, medicine is perhaps more dependent than any other on access to the current world literature for up-to-date knowledge and practice guidelines. Over the working lifetime of the professional, that knowledge must be maintained current and expanded — a daunting task for a busy professional. Current indications are that there are well over 1 million items of information relevant to medical practice, and that on a good day and under ideal conditions the average student can absorb about 7 such items each hour. Simple arithmetic reveals that working a 12 hour day for 250 days a year as a full time student, it would take nearly 50 years just to catch up with current knowledge.

Larry Weed (of PROMIS fame — see chapter 2) reflected on the changes in his thinking from the time he entered medical school, at which time he was sure that he would be able to memorise everything he would need to be a skilled clinician. Many years later he reported his perception that the skilled clinician needed to make use of technology to extend his/her memory, just as he/she made use of technology to see inside patients and to measure invisible chemicals in the blood.

Health practitioners are well aware of the availability of this knowledge in the world medical literature, and, indeed are aware that much of the more important material may even be on the bookshelves at their home, office or local library. But there is so much material and it changes so fast that learning and memorising it can prove difficult. The process of trying to keep abreast of the current literature is also potentially fraught with danger, since it is all too easy to get the details confused in a domain as broad and complex as medicine. The sheer size of the literature makes it difficult and time-consuming to locate a specific fact or reference just when it is needed: navigation of the literature is a major problem.

It is clear that the safe and successful practice of medicine must depend upon access to an integrated literature, and to abstraction of relevant knowledge from that literature. The medical literature is full of **data,** that is of experimental observations and results. Often these data items are interpreted, within the limited experimental context of the study reported, into **information,** and that information may itself be useful to practitioners. However, it generally requires review articles or textbooks to bring the information together and present it in an integrated and useable form. At this stage the information can be viewed as **knowledge** and rules for the use of that information may have been added.

However, knowledge stored on paper is still often difficult to find and fit to the situation confronting the user: it is not **dynamic.** The information may all be there on the pages, but the user cannot readily compile a synopsis of all those conditions in which a particular constellation of signs and symptoms could be present. The task of making this knowledge dynamic is well under way. The availability of information in electronic form means that it can be responsive to the specific needs of the enquirer, and can be structured, searched and presented in whatever form the user may require for that specific purpose.

Where is the information?

The biomedical literature is generally nowhere near the health professional. The literature from your viewpoint can be divided up into:

1. materials in your bookcase (texts, journals)
2. materials in a nearby library
3. materials in neither of the above locations (the vast majority)

Every individual has a personal collection of reference materials: these are especially useful because they are the works that are familiar to their owner and are therefore quick and easy to use. Many may be the texts used as a student at medical school. Each individual uses a limited number of texts in a flexible way: they memorise the contents of these volumes, and know pretty well where they will be able to find material about a specific issue. Inevitably, these reference materials are out of date and may contain practices, commentary and analyses which are not only erroneous but possibly dangerous.

Most clinicians try to keep up by reading journals and periodicals, and attending seminars and refresher courses. However, the size of the task is daunting. Important information may be skimmed when first encountered, but when it is needed the details and source have often been forgotten. A simple personal database of information resources, even one that just lists titles, journals and author, is often useful: the title is related to the content, and each journal has a niche in the biomedical information environment that it addresses specifically. Several companies provide collated lists of journal contents relating to a specific domain, such as AIDS.

There is often a local medical library, at least in major centres and institutions. However, the size and cost of the medical literature precludes most libraries from carrying more than a rather limited subset of the available world biomedical literature. Libraries catalogue their own holdings, as well as those of other associated libraries, often using sophisticated database technology that can allow the user considerable flexibility in searching. However, the library normally makes no attempt to provide an index of the specific contents of holdings, and the task of locating required information may become harder as the amount of information available increases. Navigation of the available resources becomes a limiting factor in the search for information.

Nevertheless, most local libraries can offer access to the world literature. They have publications that list resources held elsewhere, as well as indexing and abstracting the current literature (e.g. Current Contents). The rapid growth of CD-ROM technology is rapidly disseminating vast amounts of data, sometimes in full text form. The library also often has terminals that can go on-line to remote databases for further information, which give it access to the world literature. They can also normally arrange to obtain copies of material from other libraries at the request of the user.

The world literature

The entire world biomedical literature is vast, but access to it is actually becoming progressively quicker and easier. Originally there was the Index Medicus, started in 1879 by John Shaw Billings, second Director of the United States National Library of Medicine (NLM): this was conceived as a means to create a paper-based catalogue of the world literature relevant to biomedical issues. Over the intervening years the form of the index has changed, but the basic principles remain.

Currently the NLM has a collection of in excess of 4,000,000 books and monographs and subscribes to some 27,000 journals and periodicals. All of these are catalogued and organised by the library. Whilst it would be possible to make this entire catalogue available to the public, this is not the present policy, mainly because of the degradation in system performance and increased problems with use that would ensue. In practice, about 3300–3400 journals are selected from this list and are abstracted to provide the more than 12,000,000 references that are available electronically to the public through MEDLINE.

MEDLINE is just one of the computerised databases that the NLM supports in the suite comprising MEDLARS (MEDical Literature Analysis and Retrieval System): some others include

BIOETHICSLINE (bioethical information)
CANCERLIT (cancer information)
CATLINE (library catalogue)
CHEMLINE (chemical compounds)
DIRLINE (directory of information resources)
HEALTH (non-clinical aspects of health care)
HISTLINE (history of medicine)
POPLINE (population and family planning)
PDQ (Physicians Data Query related to cancer trials and treatments)
RTECS (toxic effects of chemical substances)
TOXLINE (toxicology of pharmaceuticals and chemicals)

MEDLINE covers biomedicine publications from 1966 to the present. Citations refer to non-English language materials (25 per cent) as well as those published in English. Some 20,000–25,000 new references are added each month: these can be searched separately from the main MEDLINE database under SDILINE (Selective Dissemination of Information), to avoid the waste associated with repetitive searching of the main database itself.

How does MEDLINE work?

Almost everyone is familiar with the traditional card index systems that are used by libraries. These organise entries into a defined order, based upon (1) the name of the author and/or (2) the subject matter and title of the publication.

These card index catalogues refer only to books and monographs: although each journal is recorded, there is no attempt to catalogue the diverse contents of the periodicals and their multitude of articles. Consequently the vast bulk of the available material, and especially the current research, is hidden from library information retrieval system.

MEDLINE fills this niche. It classifies the contents of the journals, article by article, from across the world. Each article is read by library staff, and certain features of it are recorded for the database. Amongst the features recorded are:

title (in English, and original title, where translated)
author(s) (up to 10) and address
source of article (journal, volume, issue, serial number, country etc.)
abstract of article (since 1975, 400 words maximum)
subject of article

The most widely used data are also made available on an optical disk (CD-ROM) by subscription. Each disk typically holds the records for one year. Many libraries and hospitals have equipped themselves with MEDLINE on CD, and often make it available to staff throughout the institution using their local area networks.

The biggest difference between the on-line and CD versions is the speed with which new abstracts are accessible. The on-line system has all abstracts available as soon as they are entered: the CD introduces a delay of a month or two before new abstracts are distributed. During the current year, an updated CD is usually distributed to subscribers every month or thereabouts.

Searching

In searching the database the user can specify that the record be retrieved only if the field selected:

1. contains a specific entry (e.g. **Author = Smith**, so excluding Smithers or Smithson),
2. contains a predefined range of entries (e.g. **Publication Year = 1984–1987,** often specified using > < signs, (in this instance >1983&<1988))
3. contains a predefined sequence of characters (e.g. **Title contains the "string" *comput*,** so including computer, computers, microcomputer, computing, computed)

Whilst "string" searching is relatively slow, especially if the field involved is long, it may be invaluable. You might retrieve from MEDLINE all articles on the inotropic effects of digoxin using the subject classification, but then separate just those research papers based on rat studies by performing a string search of their abstracts to see if the word *rat* appeared in the abstract. MEDLINE has 23 defined fields in its structure, and each field is searchable.

You can, for example, construct a search of the form:

find	**leukopenia**	MeSH heading Leukopaenia
and	**LA=english**	limit to English LAnguage
and	**PY=1988**	limit to Publication Year 1988
and	**Br-J-Cancer in SO**	limit to SOurce is British Journal of Cancer

which will return to you 4 citations out of the 351,639 references indexed for the year 1988 (using the Silver Platter CD-ROM).

Content classification

The way in which the subject matter of journal articles is categorised and recorded deserves further study. MEDLINE (and other MEDLARS databases) use a system called Medical Subject Headings (MeSH), which is an hierarchical system, with Major Headings and Minor Headings. All references are classified using terms from MeSH by NLM indexation staff. MeSH has some 15,000 "preferred terms" with another 40,000 approximate synonyms of those terms and a further 80,000 chemical terms.

To explain the preferred terms, a search for "enlarged spleen" would be unsuccessful, because the preferred term is "splenomegaly": similarly "arthritis, rheumatoid" is the preferred term (not "rheumatoid arthritis"), and "leukopenia" is the preferred term (not low white cell count, or WBC lowered, or even leucocytopaenia). Whilst MeSH prefers US spellings, most non-US spellings of terms are recognised as synonyms.

Alternatively you could enter the term "leukopenia" and call up the Thesaurus to identify what terms are preferred and searchable related to this topic, and what dimensions can be distinguished during the search. If you do this you will find the term hierarchy:

Hemic and Lymphatic Disorders
    Leukocyte Disorders
        Leukopenia
        Agranulocytosis
        Lymphopenia

Selecting the term leukopenia from this and using the "explode" option offers 36 catalogued dimensions that can be associated with the term and which help the user to select appropriate references. For example:

BL-Blood;   CF-Cerebrospinal-fluid;   CI-Chemically-induced;
EC-Economics;   EH-Ethnology   EM-Embryology;
PP-Physiopathology;   PS-Parasitology PX-Psychology;

Knowledge bases and decision support tools

MEDLINE is a rich source of information about the biomedical sciences. However, the content is simply information: it is up to the user to consider how that information might best be applied to a specific clinical scenario.

The key to ensuring that best use is made of available information is to develop tools that encapsulate that knowledge in an easy-to-use form, as an adjunct to the clinical decision making process. The role of the care provider in this new scenario would be to gather information and make clinical observations, as well as to manage the process of the encounter and to interact productively with the patient. The computer would provide the up-to-date clinical information as and when required, and could also propose hypotheses, suggest avenues of inquiry and critique decisions. Knowledge tools of this sort are already in existence, and many more will be developed in the near future. Some examples of available knowledgebases are Quick Medical Reference (QMR), and Problem Knowledge Couplers (PKC).

Taking this a step further, it is possible for the entire patient encounter to be directed by computer software incorporating artificial intelligence (AI). Medical **expert systems** have been available for some time, and typically can perform at least as well as a skilled practitioner.

The special attraction of either of these approaches is that new knowledge can be added to the computerised information resources as it is discovered, and updates distributed immediately, ensuring minimal delays in getting that knowledge into the workplace.

Protocols used for data gathering and treatment planning are further examples of linking information with computer software to create powerful clinical tools. These guide the professional as to what information should be collected, so ensuring that all relevant information is available before a decision is made.

Use of information resources

Many health professionals are motivated to keep their knowledge up-to-date, but find it difficult in the context of a demanding work schedule. Most would at least scan the pages of one or two journals, and many would regularly attend some professional meetings and refresher courses. However, it is widely accepted that continuing medical education, as it is called, has not been successful in maintaining optimal levels of knowledge and understanding thus far. Electronic access to information has the potential to change this by reducing reliance on what the professional may have memorised, rightly or wrongly, and ensuring that appropriate, accurate and current information is always to hand, even in the most remote and backward communities.

However, use of electronic information and knowledge resources is still very limited. In part this may be because of the generally low levels of use of technology. Even where technology is used, the knowledge bases are not linked in to the medical records system and the user often has to move to another terminal or location to access the knowledge base. Attitudes towards the use of electronic information resources will change. One major pressure is that of litigation in relation to misadventures that have arisen and could have been avoided if the practitioner had made use of available knowledge resources. Ignorance of the facts in the information age is unlikely to be acceptable as a defence to a charge of professional negligence. However, it will still be a doctor who has to defend his actions in court, even if they were performed at the suggestion of an expert system.

Clinical audit

Audit is the systematic, critical analysis of the quality of care, including the appropriateness, sequence and timing of the procedures used for diagnosis and treatment, the overall consumption of resources, and the resulting outcome and quality of life for the patient. It is conducted on a case-by-case basis, usually by a dedicated audit team, and constitutes an essential activity for highlighting patterns and outcomes of care that are more or less desirable. Audit is generally seen primarily as a formative activity where constructive peer review contributes to the experiences and expertise of all involved, and to the overall performance of a service unit. However, persistent pressures to improve cost-effectiveness, service quality and unit performance may lead to the use of audit data in awarding contracts and attracting business.

The activities of any healthcare institution can be assessed in terms of:

1. the *efficiency* of production of diagnostic, therapeutic and other services, as measured by the cost or time taken to provide each service (such as a chest x-ray or a therapeutic procedure)
2. the *effectiveness* of the selection by clinicians of diagnostic, therapeutic and other services, in order to achieve the desired outcome for individual patients, with the minimum of cost, time, inconvenience and complications, and including the sequenceing and timing of services ordered and provided
3. the *quality* of services provided in terms of meeting predefined standards of quality

Some writers have tried to draw a distinction between clinical audit and medical audit, implying that clinical audit relates to all of the treatment provided to patients by a healthcare organisation, whether by doctors, nurses or paramedical staff, while medical audit covers only the work done by doctors assessed by peer review. Here the two terms are used synonymously.

Audit systems and reports

In reporting the results of audit it is often helpful to show incidence rates per 100 or per 1000 patients. However, such figures are meaningless unless the denominator, or total sample size is reliable. It is vital to ensure that data collection is complete and consistent, and that all relevant patients are audited. Audit studies which concentrate only on patients who have complications to the exclusion of straightforward cases may be misleading.

The hospital's patient administration system (PAS) routinely records admissions and discharges, and in some cases, outpatient attendances. The basic demographic (name, age, sex etc.) and episode data should be downloaded electronically from the PAS to an audit system. Such data may provide performance indicators such as time on waiting list, length of stay, post-operative stay, preoperative delay and readmission rates.

The audit computer system may generate a form for each patient to be completed either by audit assistants or by clinicians. This audit form may be a simple form with boxes to be ticked, or an optical mark readable (OMR) form, which can be read directly into the computer, saving transcription at a later stage.

The data collection process includes the identification of adverse patient events and incidents as well as a review of the quality, timeliness and completeness of documentation in the medical record. Clinical data such as principal and secondary diagnoses, diagnostic and therapeutic procedures and their practitioners also need to be collected. This may be obtained retrospectively from coded data used for hospital statistics, or preferably prospectively directly from the clinicians.

Clinical research

The procedures and systems required for clinical research are essentially the same as those outlined for audit earlier in this chapter. However, the range of data that may be required for clinical research varies widely.

Many research studies have been confounded through inappropriate use of computer systems, and in this section just some of the key issues are identified. The big problem with retrospective clinical research is that the dataset recorded for each patient varies, and the cost and difficulty of extracting the relevant data from handwritten records is prohibitive.

The three issues addressed below are generic and apply to the setting up and maintenance of any database. However they are often confronted for the first time when a clinical department decides to conduct a clinical study with all staff entering the data direct into a computerised collection system. It is for this reason that they are included here.

How much data?

Most studies are set up by enthusiasts: their enthusiasm for the study leads them to try to collect every possible item of data, whether or not it has any bearing on the current hypothesis being researched. The argument is that it just might turn out to be important, and it is much easier to collect it prospectively than retrospectively. In part the argument is correct: as stated above it is much easier to collect data prospectively. However, the whole argument is fallacious and a prime cause of failed studies.

Trying to collect everything possible about each subject has the following effects:

- prolonged data collection times which interferes with other work to be done, and often causes some distress to the subject
- staff irritation with the data collection process adding extra work for no return (to them)
- massive amounts of data to be entered and stored, leading to excessively large databases or spreadsheets, and difficulty in data manipulation

- problems with classification and coding of the data
- confusion about the real purposes of the study

Data adequacy and validation

The database is only as good as the worst information within it. The accuracy, validity (quality) and adequacy (completeness) of a dataset are crucial considerations. These are of special concern when there are several individuals gathering the data, some of whom may have precious little commitment to the goals of the study.

Adequacy — data may be collected free form or within a structured collection process. The free form data collection process is likely to be incomplete: issues will inevitably be omitted in the data collection for some subjects, thus creating incomplete data sets.

The solution to this problem is to use a proforma, either on paper (e.g. check boxes) or in electronic form. The checklist may need to be transcribed manually into a computerised database (when transcription errors may arise, affecting quality), or may be designed for direct reading by a device such as an Optical Mark Reader (OMR), which can greatly reduce errors. However, electronic data collection protocols are in most instances the best way to go. These present the questions, in sequence, and accept entries directly into the database. Branches can be invoked automatically in response to certain data entries, which ensures that no irritatingly redundant questions are asked, and no important issues are overlooked. Adequacy of data is thereby ensured. Electronic data collection also provides an opportunity to ensure data quality and validation (see below).

Validation — any data that may be used as a key for finding and sorting records must be as accurately recorded as possible. The data string entered into a record may be meaningful or meaningless: in many cases the meaningless data arises as a result of a keystroke error (remember 1 in 20 keystrokes on average are erroneous). For example, where data is coded (see below), some codes may be valid and others invalid having no assigned meaning. Where data entry is carried out electronically, entries can be checked at the time to ensure that they are valid values: invalid entries can be rejected then and there and a prompt displayed seeking a correction. This on-line validation does not ensure that the code entered is accurate, but at least ensures that nonsense entries are eliminated.

A typical example would be recording of resting pulse rate. The normal range might be defined as 60–125 beats/minute, with figures outside this range triggering a warning to the operator to check the entry. The system might be further programmed to refuse to accept entries outside the range of 40–200 beats/min as being impossible. Similarly the codes 1–5 might have been assigned to describe pulse rates that are *very low, low, normal, high or very high*: an entry of 6,7,8 or 9 would be rejected as meaningless or invalid data. Validation of text entries is handled in just the same way: unless the string entered matches exactly a valid value stored in a table, the entry is rejected. The process can be facilitated through the use of "picking lists" where the first few characters entered bring up a list of valid values from which the user can select that which is appropriate using a pointer.

Measuring outcomes

Three classes of outcome measure have been developed — health profiles, specific indicator measures and global measures.

Health profiles tend to be long checklists or questionaires covering a large number of health-related items. These are suited to research studies where there is plenty of time to collect and analyse large amounts of data on a limited number of patients.

Specific indicator measures are normally diagnosis, treatment or specialty specific, designed to measure progress for a specific condition. Much clinical research uses such measures. Disadvantages of indicator measures are:

- impossibility of making comparisons between patients suffering from different conditions
- inability to account for patients having multiple problems
- focus on the disease process, not the whole patient.

Global outcome measures are designed to measure the outcome of healthcare on a common basis, applicable to all patients irrespective of what is the matter with them, in order to permit comparisons between specialties and casemix groups.

Selected bibliography

This bibliography has been restricted to books and articles in key journals which are readily available from most libraries.

Abbott W (ed) (1991) *Information Technology in Health Care: A Handbook* Longman, Harlow

Bakker A R *et al* (eds) (1988) *Towards New Hospital Information Systems* North Holland, Amsterdam

Ball M J *et al* (eds) (1988) *Nursing Informatics: Where Caring and Technology Meet* Springer-Verlag, New York

Bardsley M, Coles J and Jenkins L (eds) (1988) *DRGs and healthcare: the management of case mix* Kings Fund, London

Benson T J R (1978) *Classification of Disability and Distress* by Ward Nurses: a Reliability Study *Int J Epidemiol*, 359–361

Benson T J R (1982) Computers in General Practice *RCGP Reference Book* 395–396, London.

Benson T J R (1989) The Challenge of Standardised Terminology in the Health Field in Scherrer J R, Cote R A and Mandil S H (eds) *Computerised Natural Medical Language Processing for Knowledge Representation*, 41–45 North Holland, Amsterdam

Benson T J R (1990) Health Cards — The Move Towards Standards *Smart Card Monthly*, April, 11–13

Benson T J R DRGs are coming *British Journal of Healthcare Computing* (7) 2, 27–28

Benson T J R (1991) *Medical Informatics: A Report for Managers and Clinicians* Longman Health Services Management, Harlow

Benson T J R (1993) *Doctors, Managers and Computers* NHS-CCC, Loughborough

Benson T J R And Twaites E (1987) Reasons to Computerise Pathology. Supplement to the *British Journal of Healthcare Computing*, iii-v

Blois M (1984) *Information and Medicine: The Nature of Medical Descriptions* University of California Press

Blum B (1986) *Clinical Information Systems* Springer-Verlag, New York

Blum B I and Duncan K (eds) (1990) *A History of Medical Informatics* ACM Press, New York

Brewer M (1982) *Information Security* DISC Management Guide, BSI, London

Bright R (1988) *Smart Cards: Principles, Practice, Applications* Ellis Horwood, Chichester

Carr R C (1992) *Document Interchange* DISC Management Guide, BSI, London

CCTA (1991) *GOSIP V4.0 Government OSI Profile* HMSO, London

CEN TC251 (1994) *Directory of European Standardisation Requirements for Healthcare Informatics and Programme for the Development of Standards* CEN, Brussels

Chard T (1988) *Computing for Clinicians* Elmore-Chard, London

Clough B and Mungo P (1992) *Approaching Zero: Computer Crime and the Computer Underworld* Faber and Faber, London

Coad P and Yourdon E (1991) *Object-Oriented Analysis* Prentice-Hall, Englewood Cliffs NJ

Cook H and Garside P (eds) (1993) *Managing NHS Trusts* Longman Health Management, Harlow

Cote R A (ed) (1984) *SNOMED Systematized Nomenclature of Medicine* College of American Pathologists, Skokie

CR 1350 (1993) *Investigation of Syntaxes for Existing Interchange Formats to be used in Healthcare* CEN, Brussels

De Dombal T (1993) *Surgical Decision Making* Butterworth Heinemann, Oxford

De Moor G. et. al. (eds) (1993) *Progress in Standardization in Health Care Informatics* IOS Press, Amsterdam

Department of Health (1990) *GP Computing: Information for GPs on Practices Computer Systems* HMSO, London

Dick R S and Steen E B (eds) (1991) *The Computer-based Patient Record: An Essential Technology for Health Care* National Academy Press, Washington

Duisterhout J et. al. (eds) (1991) *Telematics in Medicine* North Holland, Amsterdam

Dixon N (1991) *Medical Audit Primer* Healthcare Quality Quest, Romsey

Drummond M F, Stoddart G L and Torrance G W (eds) (1987) *Methods for the Economic Evaluation of Healthcare Programmes* Oxford Medical Publications, Oxford

Ellis D (1987) *Medical Computing and Applications* Ellis Horwood, Chichester

Evans C R (1979) *The Mighty Micro: The Impact of the Computer Revolution* Victor Gollancz, London

ENV 1068 (1993) *Medical Informatics — Healthcare Information Interchanges — Registration of Coding Schemes* CEN, Brussels

EWOS (1991) *Medical Data Interchange: Final Report of EWOS PT007* EWOS, Brussels

Fetter R B *et al* (1980) Case-Mix Definition by Diagnosis Related Groups *Medical Care* (18) 1–53

Fetter R B (1988) Information Systems Requirements for Case Mix Management by DRG in Bakker A R et. al. (eds) *Towards New Hospital Information Systems*, 161–167 North Holland, Amsterdam

Fitchett T (1992) *Network Management* DISC Management Guide, BSI, London

General Medical Services Committee (1990) *Guidance to General Medical Practitioners on Data Protection Registration* BMA, London

Harrington J J, Benson T J R and Spector A (1990) IEEE P1157 Medical data interchange (MEDIX) committee: overview and status report in Miller R A (ed) *SCAMC Proceedings*, 230–234, IEEE Computer Society Press

Health Level Seven (1994) *HL7 Version 2.2* Chicago, Illinois

Herbert S I, Molteno B W H, Ashford J R and Cumming G (1982) *A Time for Decision? Computing Policy and Practice in the NHS* Nuffield Provincial Hospitals Trust, London

Hopkins A (1990) *Measuring the Quality of Medical Care* Royal College of Physicians, London

Hopkins R J (1990) The Exeter Care Card Project *HC90 Proceedings*, 236–242 BJHC Books, Weybridge

Houldsworth J (1992) Open Systems DISC Management Guide, BSI, London

Hugo I (1991) *Practical Open Systems: A Guide for Managers* NCC Blackwell, Oxford

Hunt J W (1992) *Managing People at Work: A Manager's Guide to Behaviour in Organisations* McGraw-Hill, London

ICD-10 (1992) *International Statistical Classification of Diseases and Related Health Problems: Tenth Revision* WHO, Geneva

Irvine D and Irvine S (eds) (1991) *Making Sense of Audit* Radcliffe Medical Press, Oxford

ISO 5281 (1977) *Information Interchange — Representation of Human Sexes* ISO, Geneva

ISO 7498 (1984) Information Processing Systems — Open Systems Interconnection — Basic Reference Model

ISO 9735 (1992) *Electronic Data Interchange for Administration Commerce and Transport (EDIFACT) - Application Level Syntax Rules* ISO, Geneva

King Taylor L (1992) *Quality: Total Customer Service* Century Business, London

Korner E (ed) (1982) *Steering Group on Health Services Information: First Report* HMSO, London

Lamberts H and Wood M (eds) (1987) *ICPC International Classification of Primary Care* Oxford Medical Publications, Oxford

Lindley D (1971) *Making Decisions* Wiley-Interscience, London

Lucas R W, Knill-Jones R P, Card W I and Crean G P (1976) Computer Interrogation of Patients *Brit Med J*, 2, 623–625

Malcolm A and Poyser J (eds) (1982) *Computers and the General Practitioner* Pergamon Press, Oxford

Marinker M (ed) (1990) Medical Audit and General Practice *Brit Med J*, London

Markwell D C (1990) Patient Held Medical Record in Communication Strategy *HC90 Proceedings*, 136–142 BJHC Books, Weybridge

McDonald C J (1990) Standards for the Electronic Transfer of Clinical Data: Progress, Promises and the Conductors Wand in Miller R A (ed) *SCAMC Proceedings*, 9–14, IEEE Computer Society Press

McDonald C J (1984) The search for national standards for medical data interchange *MD Computing*; (1)1:3–4

Meyer B (1988) *Object-oriented Software Construction* Prentice Hall, New York

Neame R (1990) Keeping an Open Mind *Health Service Journal*, 1077–1080

NHS Management Executive (1990) *The Care Card: Evaluation of the Exmouth Project* HMSO, London

NHS Management Executive (1991) *NHS Data Manual* Information Management Group, Stanmore

NHS Management Executive (1992) *Getting better with Information: Handbook for IMBT Specialists* IMG External Communications Office, Cambridge

NHS Management Executive (1992) *Information Systems Security* NHS IMC Birmingham

NHS Management Executive (1993) *General Medical Practice Computer Systems: Requirements for Accreditation* IMG, Leeds.

NHS Management Executive (1993) *Hospital Systems Report 1993, A Report on the Implementation of Hospitals Information Systems in England* IMG, Leeds

Noothoven van Goor J and Christensen J P (eds) (1992) *Advances in Medical Informatics: Results of the AIM Exploratory Action* IOS Press, Amsterdam

Perry J (1978) *Oxmis Problem Codes* Oxford Community Health Project, Oxford

Pollock A and Evans M (1993) *Surgical Audit* Butterworth-Heinemann, London

Preece J (1990) *The Use of Computers in General Practice* Churchill Livingstone, Edinburgh

Pye C (1988) *What is OSI?* NCC Publications, Manchester

Rea C (1993) *Managing Clinical Directorates* Longman Health Management, Harlow

Read J D and Benson T J R (1986) Comprehensive Coding *British Journal of Healthcare Computing* 3 (2) [May] 22–25

Richards B (ed) (1994) HC 94: *Current Perspectives in Healthcare Computing* Conference Proceedings, BJHC, Weybridge

Ritchie L D (1985) *Computers in Primary Care* Heinemann

Roger-France F H *et al* (eds) (1989) Diagnosis Related Groups in Europe *UZ-Dienst Medische Informatica*, Gent

Rosser R M and Watts V C (1972) The Measurement of Hospital Output *Int J Epidemiol* (1) 361–368

Rosser R M and Benson T J R (1978) New Tools for Evaluation: Their Application to Computers MIE 78 Proceedings, Berlin, 1–10

Rosser R M (1983) History of the Development of Health Indicators in Teeling Smith G (ed) *Measuring the Social Benefits of Medicine*, 5–62 Office of Health Economics, London

Royal College of Physicians (1989) *Medical Audit: A First Report, What, Why and How?* The Royal College of Physicians of London

Royal College of Surgeons of England (1991) *Guidelines for Surgical Audit by Computer* Royal College of Surgeons, London

Sager N, Friedman C and Lyman M S (1987) *Medical Language Processing: Computer Management of Narrative Data* Addison-Wesley, Reading MA

Scherrer J R, Cote R A and Mandil S H (eds) (1989) *Computerised Natural Medical Language Processing for Knowledge Representation* North Holland, Amsterdam

Shaw C (1990) *Medical Audit: A Hospital Handbook* King's Fund Centre, London

Shneiderman B (1987) *Designing the User Interface: Strategies for Effective Human-Computer Interaction* Addison-Wesley, Reading MA

Shortliffe E H and Perreault L E (eds) (1990) *Medical Informatics: Computer Applications in Health Care* Addison-Wesley, Reading MA

Siemasko F (ed) (1978) *Computing in Clinical Laboratories* Pitman Medical, Tunbridge Wells

SITPRO (1991) *EDIFACT Service* SITPRO, London

Slack W V, Hicks G P and Reed C E *et al* (1966) A Computer Based Medical History System *The New Eng J Med*, 274 (4), 194–198

Smith R (ed) (1992) *Audit in Action* British Medical Journal, London

Steele D (1992) *Human Computer Interaction* DISC Management Guide, BSI, London

Stevens G (1988) Selecting Computer Software Packages — A Self Help Guide *J Roy Soc Med*, Vol 81, 458–460

Stokes A V (1991) *OSI Standards and Acronyms* NCC Blackwell, Manchester

Teeling Smith G (ed) (1983) *Measuring The Social Benefits of Medicine* Office of Health Economics, London

Tyndall R *et al* (1990) *Computers in Medical Audit: A Guide for Hospital Consultants to Personal Computer (PC) Based Medical Audit Systems* Royal Society of Medicine Services, London

Weed L L (1969) *Medical Records, Medical Education and Patient Care: The Problem Oriented Record as a Basic Tool* Year Book Medical Publishers, Chicago

Weed L L (1990) The Premises and Tools of Medical Care and Medical Education: Perspectives Over 40 Years in Blum B I and Duncan K (eds) *A History of Medical Informatics*, 222–249 ACM Press, New York

Weed L L (1991) *Knowledge Coupling: New Premises and New Tools for Medical Care and Education* Springer-Verlag, New York

Winograd T and Flores F (1987) *Understanding Computers and Cognition: A New Foundation for Design* Addison-Wesley, Reading MA

Glossary and acronyms

4GL Fourth generation language — A programming environment which permits rapid software development and maintenance

ADT Admission, Discharge and Transfer — A patient administration system for inpatients

AIM Advanced Informatics in Medicine — The European research and development programme in healthcare computing

ALGORITHM A precise statement of a method of calculation or working out a problem. It can sometimes be expressed conveniently in a programming language.

ANALOGUE Representation of entities based on relative value, e.g. intensity of colour, pitch of a sound (cf digital).

ANSI American National Standards Institute

ARCHITECTURE A framework from which applications, databases and workstations can be developed in a coherent manner, and in which every part fits together without containing a mass of design details.

ARGUMENT The part of a command line that specifies what the command is to do.

ASCII American Standard Code for Information Interchange — Many computers store characters internally using a special code called ASCII. The computer sorts alphanumeric characters into ascending ASCII order. ASCII code is the only universally agreed code for data exchange, but much detail is lost (e.g. page layout details) during such exchange since ASCII has no codes for these entities.

ASTM — American Society for Testing and Materials — One of the US standards bodies.

AUDIT — Medical audit is the systematic critical analysis of the quality of medical care including the procedures used for diagnosis and treatment, the use of resources and the resulting outcome and quality of life for the patient.

AVAILABILITY — One of the security requirements — availability, integrity and confidentiality. Availability indicates that the computing services are functional and accessible to (authorised) users as and when they are required.

BACKGROUND PROCESS — A secondary process which runs concurrently but "behind" the principal process appearing on the computer terminal. A process that is active but normally unseen by the user.

BACKUP — A copy of a file or disk. Making copies of software and/or data in case the original is lost, corrupted, or destroyed is referred to as "backing up"

BAUD RATE — The number of bits per second passing a communications channel.

BATCH MODE — A non-interactive mode of using a computer, in which users submit jobs for processing and receive results later on completion.

BENCHMARK — A program or programs designed to test the speed and power of a computer. The values obtained are usually based on performance of an arithmetic task, and may not relate directly to practical applications. They provide only a rough guide for comparing the performance of one computer against another.

BINARY — A numbering system to base 2, rather than the base 10 commonly used. Only two binary digits exist, 0 and 1. This can be represented in a computer by a simple switch (off = 0, on = 1).

BIT	A binary digit that can assume the values of either 0 or 1. (See also Byte). An entry processed by a digital computer is reduced to a sequence of bits (See ASCII).
BOOT	The process of starting up the computer, that is, loading the operating system, derived from the phrase "pulling one's self up by the boot straps".
BOOTABLE DISK	A floppy disk containing part of the operating system which allows the computer to boot. If you ever need to reformat your hard disk you need a bootable disk.
BROADBAND	A transmission medium with a high capacity for information transfer.
BSI	British Standards Institution — BSI represents British interests on all international standards organisations such as CEN and ISO.
BUFFER	A temporary store of data. For example, data waiting to be printed is held in a print buffer.
BUG	An error or malfunction in a computer or piece of software.
BUS	A distribution system for data. The bus links hardware elements together (e.g within a PC or in a Local Area Network (LAN)). The bus specification lays down which pins on the connectors serve which functions.
BYTE	The computer stores information as a series of bits electrical off and on switches (binary form). Eight bits comprise one "byte"; and one byte is sufficient to represent one keyboard character (See ASCII). The storage capacity of computer memory is measured in kilobytes (Kb) or megabytes (Mb). 1 Kb is 2^{10} or 1024 bytes and 1 Mb is 2^{20} or 1048576 bytes.
CCC	NHS Centre for Coding and Classification — The NHS CCC is responsible for the development of the Read Codes.
CCITT	Comite Consultatif International Telegraphique et Telephonique, the international body responsible for telecommunications standards.

CD-ROM	Compact Disk — Read-Only Memory — A means of storage large amounts of data (typically >600 Mb) in a compact format which is read by a laser device.
CEN	Comite Europeen de Normalisation — The main European standards organisation.
CEN TC251	The CEN Technical Committee responsible for standards in healthcare computing.
CENELEC	Comite Europeen de Normalisation Electrotechnique — CENELEC is the European body responsible for standards relating to electrical and electronic devices, e.g. operating theatre equipment.
CHARACTER	A printable symbol such as "A" or "," or "3" etc.
CHARACTER STRING	A sequence of characters which may contain letters, numbers, punctuation characters or blank spaces. "Abies MIS Ltd" is a character string.
CHIP	An integrated circuit containing a number of miniaturised electronic devices. CPU chips today contain more than 5,000,000 separate transistors in a single package.
CIS	Clinical Information System used by clinicians.
CISC	Complex Instruction Set Computer. (See also RISC).
CLASSIFI-CATION	Classification is the systematic placement of things or concepts into categories which share some common attribute, quality or property.
CLIENT SERVER	System architecture where the user works on a workstation (client) using data held on a remote database (server).
CLNS	Connectionless-mode Network Service used on local area networks (e.g. Ethernet).
CLOCK SPEED	This measure, referred to in MHz (mega-Hertz), is an indicator of the speed with which a processor can execute instructions.

CODE | A fixed sequence of signs or symbols, alphabetic or numeric characters, serving to designate an object or a concept.

CODING SCHEME | A system for classifying objects and entities (such as diseases, procedures or symptoms) using a finite set of numeric or alphanumeric identifiers.

COMMAND | A sequence of words and/or symbols that instruct the computer to perform a specific task. Normally followed by an argument that indicates the object (e.g file) to which the command is to be applied.

COMPATIBILITY | The property that enables two different systems to be connected and work together for specific practical purposes.

COMPILER | A program that translates a program written in a high-level programming language to a machine-language program, which can then be executed.

COMPUTER SYSTEM | An integrated arrangement of computer hardware and software, operated by users to perform prescribed tasks.

CONFIDEN-TIALITY | An element of security (see also Availability and Integrity). Access to stored data is restricted to those with specific authority to view the data.

CONFORM-ANCE TESTING | The testing of devices claimed to conform to certain standards to establish whether they actually do so.

CONS | Connection-Oriented Network Service used on wide area networks (e.g. X.25).

CONTROL CHARACTER | A special character that is interpreted by the computer for a special task. For example, CONTROL-D is used in UNIX to signal the end of a process. Often represented using the "hat" symbol, e.g. ^D.

CONTROL KEY | A key that is used in the same manner as the shift key to impart a different meaning to letter keys on the keyboard. Often represented in text as "<CTRL>".

CPT-4	Current Procedural Terminology — This coding scheme is used in the US as a guide to services for which patients may be billed.
CPU	Central Processing Unit — the "heart" of a computer where instructions are executed.
CSMA/CD	Carrier-Sense Multiple Access/Collision Detection — a network protocol which provides for recovery from message collisions on CLNS networks.
CT SCAN	Computerised Tomography — a technique of creating sectional views of the internal structure of an entity (e.g. a human body) by combining multiple images made using x-rays projected from different directions.
CURSOR	A marker or pointer generated by the program on the screen. It is represented by a small flashing block (or dot or underscore) and can be moved around using the Enter, Backspace or direction keys, or the mouse.
DATABASE	A collection of stored data — typically organised into fields, records and files — and an associated description (schema).
DATUM (plural DATA)	Any single item or fact. A medical datum generally can be regarded as the value of a specific parameter (for example, red-blood-cell count) for a particular object (for example, a patient) at a specific time often measured in a specific way.
DECRYPTION	The process of obtaining a clear message from an encrypted message.
DECISION SUPPORT	Provision of information relevant to the context of the decision maker.
DEFAULT	The action the computer takes if no further information is provided. An assumed value or instruction. For example, an instruction to manipulate a file assumes, as a default (that is unless otherwise stated) that the file is located in the present working directory.
DELIMIT	To mark or set off. For example the day, month and year values in a data string, e.g. 2/8/89 are delimited by the "/" symbol.

DHA	District Health Authority
DIAGNOSIS	The cause of a patient's problem. Various qualifiers such as provisional, working, primary, secondary, admitting, are applied to diagnosis. A differential diagnosis is a list of plausible possibilities as to the cause.
DIGITAL	Representation of an entity based on binary (on/off) signals.
DIN	Deutsches Institut fur Normung — The German national standards organisation.
DIRECTORY	A collection of files contained in the same subdivision of a disk.
DISC	A group within the BSI (Delivering Information Standards to Customers). DISC is responsible for information technology standards within BSI.
DISCHARGE NOTE	A brief synopsis prepared at discharge of the decisions and care services provided to a patient whilst in hospital.
DISK	A disk is used to store the computer's information. Information is recorded on a disk in a similar way to that used for recording sound on audio cassettes. The information is arranged in a series of concentric circular tracks ("cylinders") which are each divided into a number of sectors.
DISK DRIVE	Computers usually have two or three disk drives. The mechanism which rotates the disk, records the information on them and reads (replays) it back is the disk drive.
DISPLAY	The image displayed on a screen or other display device.
DOS	Disk Operating System — the most widely used microcomputer operating system.
DRG	Diagnosis Related Group — a system for classifying patient care episodes into groups which have similar implication for resource consumption, length of stay and care complexity required.

DRIVER	Software required to convert the output of a computer into the format expected by a peripheral of a specific type.
ECG	Electrocardiogram — a recording of the electrical activity of the heart.
EDI	Electronic Data Interchange — based on the electronic sending and receiving of messages.
EDIFACT	Electronic Data Interchange for Administration, Commerce and Transport — a set of rules and syntax for EDI maintained by the UN.
EDITOR	A program to add, change or delete the contents of electronic text or document files.
EPROM	Erasable Programmable Read-Only Memory (see also ROM). The erase function may not be easy to use and may require special technology.
EEPROM	Electronically Erasable Programmable Read-Only Memory (see also ROM).
EFMI	European Federation of Medical Informatics
EISA	Extended Industry Standard Architecture — a bus design used in some microcomputers.
EMULATION	The ability of a device to behave with the parameters of another device.
EN	Norme Europeene (European Standard) — a standard specification that normally takes precedence in the EC over local or national standards.
ENCRYPTION	The process of making a message unreadable other than to a recipient who has a specific key.
ENV	Europaische Vornorm (European Pre-standard) — a standard that has yet to be put into a final and definitive form for approval as EN.
EPONYM	The use of a person's name to describe an entity.
ESCAPE	A special key (ESC) or control character used to send instructions to devices (e.g. printers) on

special functions. The (ESC) key may also "kill" programs that are currently active.

ETHERNET	A protocol for local area networks, based on a CSMA/CD (Carrier-sense Multiple Access/ Collision Detection). The associated protocols have been subjected to standardisation as IEEE 802.3.
EUCLIDES	European Clinical Laboratory Data Exchange Standards (AIM project)
EWOS	European Workshop on Open Systems — a forum for open systems development.
EXECUTE	To run a program.
EXPANSION SLOTS	Connection slots within the box of the computer which allow extra hardware to be added on.
EXPERT SYSTEM	A program that provides the kind of problem analysis and advice that an expert might provide.
FDDI	Fibre Distributed Data Interface — an interface to an optical transmission medium (optical fibre).
FIELD	The smallest named unit of data in a database. Fields are grouped together to form records.
FILE	A collection of electronic data. A file has a name by which it is known to the computer, and may contain, for example, data, records, text, instructions, etc.
FILE EXTENSION	A group of characters appended to the end of a disk file name. File extensions are usually delimited from the filename with a dot (.) and contain up to 3 characters, e.g. FILENAME.TXT.
FILE FORMAT	The structure within which a computer file is recorded.
FILE SERVER	A computer dedicated to providing access to files and databases across a network.
FLOPPY DISK	A floppy plastic disk coated with a magnetic surface material that allows data to be stored in series of concentric tracks. Floppy disks are commonly found in two sizes, 5.25" and 3.5".

FLOWSHEET   A tabular summary of information that is arranged to display the values of variables as they change over time.

FORMAT   A disk must be formatted before data can be stored on it. Disks are organised as a series of compartments, called sectors, into which information is written and from which it is recalled. When you first take a new disk there is nothing at all recorded on it and before it may be used, the sectors must be magnetically marked out on the surface of the disk. This is called formatting. It is analogous to drawing lines on a piece of paper before writing on it.

FREE TEXT   Unstructured, uncoded representation of information in text format; for example, sentences describing the results of a patient's physical examination.

FTAM   File Transfer, Access and Management — a protocol for exchange of files across a communications network.

FUNCTION KEYS   A set of keys on the keyboard in addition to the usual alphanumeric keys (e.g F1, F2 etc). These are often used by programs to allow complex functions to be executed by a single keystroke (see "Macros").

GATEWAY   A mechanism (hardware and/or software) that allows access between two networks working to different protocols, or representing data in different ways.

GOSIP   Government OSI Profile — a profile of standards selected from the OSI specification.

GUI   Graphical User Interface — a way of enabling a user to interact with a computer system based on pictorial representations (icons), and usually controlled by a "point and click" device, such as a mouse.

HARD COPY   The printed output on paper from a computer.

HARD DISK   A hard disk or Winchester comprises one or more rigid disks which are not removable and are permanently sealed. The information held on a hard disk can be accessed 10 times as fast as from a floppy disk. Hard disks typically hold from 20 Mb to more than 1000 Mb of data.

HARDWARE	The physical equipment of a computer system, including the central processing unit, data-storage devices, terminals and printers.
HCP	Health Care Professional
HIS	Hospital Information System
HISPP	Health Informatics Standards Planning Panel — a body designed to oversee the development of standards in North America.
HL7	Health Level Seven — an interactive data exchange protocol for healthcare.
HMO	Health Maintenance Organisation — an organisation (in USA) purchasing care services for its members, usually through a series of clinics and facilities affiliated with or owned by the organisation.
HOMONYM	One term having two or more independent meanings.
HRG	Health Resource Group — one of the many approaches to grouping patients on the basis of similar resource implications for care.
ICD	International Classification of Disease — a classification system for causes of mortality and morbidity suited to secondary (hospital) care event reporting. Version 10 of ICD is available although most institutions are still using ID9.
ICD9CM	Clinical modifications made to the basic ICD-9 coding system. In large part, these provide for coding of procedures.
ICHPPC	International Classification of Health Problems in Primary Care
IC-Process-PC	International Classification of Process in Primary Care
ICPC	International Classification of Primary Care

ICON	A pictorial representation of an object or function in a graphical interface. A user can point to an icon and click on it to initiate that function.
ICU	Intensive Care Unit — a unit providing high intensity care for critically ill patients.
ID	Identification Details
IEC	International Electrotechnical Commission — an international standards organisation.
IEEE	Institute of Electrical and Electronic Engineers — a USA standards making body.
IMACS	Image Management and Communication Systems
IMAGING MODALITY	Definition of the technique used in production of a (clinical) image. Examples are photography, X-ray imaging, computed tomography (CT scan), echosonography (echo scan), and magnetic resonance imaging (NMR scan) as well as PET scan, thermal, j scan . . . .
IMC	NHS Information Management Centre Group
IMG	NHS Information Management Group
IMIA	International Medical Informatics Associations — a federation of such associations worldwide
INFORMATION	An assembly of organised data that provides a basis for making a decision or drawing an inference.
INPATIENT	A patient who is (temporarily) resident in a care facility.
INTEGRITY	An element of security (see also Availability, Confidentiality). All parts of the system are operating correctly according to specification and in the way the current user believes them to be operating.
INTERFACE	A common boundary between two associated systems across which information may flow. The interface may filter or modify data as it passes across the boundary.

INTERNET	The international network of computers providing support for data exchange and Email.
INTEROPER-ABILITY	The ability of systems of different architectures to pass data and commands to one another.
IOM	Institute of Medicine — a USA organisation for the advancement of medicine.
IP	In Patient — a patient who is temporarily resident in a care institution, e.g. a hospital.
ISAC	Image Save and Carry — a proposed standard for recording health data on MOD (magnetic-optical disk)
ISDN	Integrated Services Digital Network — a telecommunications network service.
ISO	International Standards Organisation — the body overseeing endorsement and publication of international standards.
IT	Information Technology
LAN	Local Area Network. A method of connecting computers together so they can share facilities, such as hard disks, data, printers etc.
LOGIN	The process where a user identifies themselves as an authorised user of a computer system.
LOGOUT	The process of exiting from the computer and terminating the current session.
MACRO	A sequence of manoeuvres that have been linked together and can be effected by a single keystroke.
MAINFRAME	A large multi-user computer, typically operated and maintained by professional computing personnel.
MBDS	Minimum Basic Data Set — a set of data required for administration purposes.
MEDICAL RECORDS	The records of care encounters, interviews and events relating to a specific patient. These include notes and letters written by doctors, nurses and

others, as well as laboratory results, clinical images, discharge notes and other materials.

MEDICAL INFORMATICS	A field of study concerned with the broad range of issues in the management and use of biomedical information, including medical computing and the study of medical information itself.
MEDINFO	The triennial world congress of medical informatics organised by IMIA.
MEDIX	Medical Data Interchange Committee (IEEE P1157) — a standards committee
MEDLINE	An on-line system providing access to the world biomedical literature through the NLM in USA.
MEMORY	The part of the system unit which holds program instructions and information being processed. This is sometimes referred to as RAM (Random Access Memory). The computer loses the information contained in the memory when the system is switched off.
MENU	A set of options listed on the screen for the user to choose from. They are usually labelled and you are asked to press the key corresponding to your choice, or to move the highlight bar to your selection.
MeSH	Medical Subject Headings — the classification system used by the NLM for indexing and navigation of the biomedical literature.
MESSAGE	Information sent by one person (computer) to another. Messages have to be structured and formatted according to a specification (syntax and semantics). The message has three parts: header, body and trailer.
MFLOPS	Millions of Floating Point Operations Per Second. A measure of the speed of a processor.
MHS	Message Handling Systems — a protocol for exchange of Email messages.
MICROWAVE	A broad band medium for the transmission of information using radio frequency waves.

MIPS	Millions of Instructions Per Second — a measure of the speed of a processor.
MOD	Magneto Optical Disk — a high capacity (c.500 Mb) erasable disk.
MODEM	MOdulator-DEModulator; A device for connecting a computer to an analogue (e.g. telephone) line for exchange of data. Modulation is a technique for carrying one or more channels of data using a base frequency as the carrier.
MODULATION	A technique for carrying one "message" signal by adding it to another "carrier" signal. The combined signal is transmitted and the message signal retrieved at the destination by subtraction of the carrier. Modulation permits low frequency signals to be broadcast effectively and is the basis for frequency division multiplexing.
MONITOR	A device for displaying text and images generated by your computer, also known as a VDU (Visual Display Unit) or screen. Current models are mainly similar to televisions, but newer displays are flat screen and based on liquid crystal devices (LCDs).
MULTIPLEX	A technique of increasing the bandwith of a transmission medium by sharing (e.g. a communications channel). Divided up on the basis either of time (time division multiplexing) where the channel is time shared by rapid switching between users, or frequency (frequency division multiplexing).
MULTI-TASKING	Multi-tasking means that the operating system can allow a user to perform more than one task at a time.
MULTI-USER	A multi-user operating system is capable of supporting more than one user at the same time.
NETWORK	An environment where many computers are linked together so as to share resources and data.
NLM	National Library of Medicine in USA — part of the US Dept of Health and Human Services. Responsible for MEDLINE.

NODE
One of the interconnected computers or devices linked in a communications network.

NOMEN-CLATURE
A nomenclature is a list of approved terms used in a technical area.

NOSOLOGY
Scientific discipline concerned with development of medical classification systems.

NUA
Network User Address — the electronic address of an individual which is assumed (temporarily) by any workstation that s/he uses to connect to that network.

NUMERIC KEYPAD
A group of keys which allow rapid entry of numerical information.

ODA
Open/Office Document Architecture — a standard format for documents.

ODIF
Open/Office Document Interchange Format — a standard for electronic exchange of ODA documents.

OFF-LINE
Equipment (e.g. printer) that can be, but is not at this moment functionally connected to the computer.

ON-LINE
Equipment that is electrically connected to and directly accessible by the computer system.

OPEN SYSTEM
Open systems are those that conform to internationally agreed standards defining computing and communication environments. These allow users to develop, run and interconnect applications and the hardware they run on, from whatever source, with minimal conversion cost. (See OSI).

OPERATING SYSTEM
A set of program routines which provide for the "housekeeping" needs of a computer, for example, relating to access disk, keyboard, screen and printer. The operating system is the first loaded when you start up your system. It stays in the system memory while you run other programs, controlling them and providing them with services.

OPTICAL DISK — A round, flat plate of plastic or metal that is used to store information. Data are encoded through the use of a laser that marks the surface of the disk, or in some other way causes a localised change of state that can be subsequently detected.

OPCS — Office of Population Censuses and Surveys — responsible for classification of procedures in UK.

OSI — Open Systems Interconnection — a set of standards for enabling connections to be made between computers regardless of their manufacturer or operating system.

OUTCOME MEASURE — A parameter for evaluating the success of an intervention.

PACKET SWITCHING — A method of passing information between any two points in a network in units (packets). The information to be passed is disassembled into packets on entry into the network, and packets then proceed individually by any available route to their destination. Before leaving the network, the packets are reassembled into their original form.

PACS — Picture Archiving and Communication System — a mechanism for electronic management of images.

PAD — Packet Assembler/Disassembler — a device required for packet-switched network connections.

PARALLEL PORT — A multicore connection between a computer and any external device that transmits data a byte (8 bits) at a time along eight wires (one bit via each wire). This produces a fast mode of transmission. However the length of the wire over which transmission can take place is limited. (See also Serial Port).

PAS — Patient Administration System (ADT)

PASSWORD — A secret word or character sequence used to identify a user to the computer system.

PATH — A route describing the relationship of a directory or file of interest to the root directory of the memory device.

PATH NAME | The absolute path name is the complete file name consisting of the file name and all directory names between the file and the root directory. The relative path name is the name of the file and all directory names between the file and the user's current working directory.

PABX | Private Automatic Branch Exchange — a telephone switchboard.

PC | Personal Computer

PERIPHERALS | Extra equipment external to the computer proper (e.g. printer, modem etc).

PIN | Personal Identification Number — a password to identify an individual to a computer system

PIPE | A process of sequencing computer commands so that the output of one command is automatically forwarded to become the input to the succeeding command.

PIXEL | One of the small picture elements that makes up a digital image. The number of pixels per square inch determines the resolution. Pixels can be associated with a single bit to indicate black and white or with multiple bits to indicate colour or grey scale.

PLATFORM | A general term for a combination of hardware and system software.

PORT | Another name for an interface. Commonly used to refer to the actual plug on the computer used to make the connection.

PORTABILITY | The ability of a program developed in one environment to be run on systems with different architectures.

PORTING | Moving software and data files to other computer systems.

PREFERRED TERM | Term recommended by an authoritative body. Normally a term that has been used for indexing a database or classification system.

PRINTER | A device for printing material onto paper.

PRIVACY	The right of individuals to control or influence who knows what about them, what information related to them may be collected and stored and by whom and to whom that information may be disclosed.
PROCESS	The computer operations or tasks initiated by a command.
PROFILE	Standards contain a large number of (combinations of) parameters (e.g. OSI). A profile is a set of selected parameters that describe a particular implementation of a standard (e.g. GOSIP).
PROGRAM	A set of instructions which can be recognised by a computer system and used to execute a set of processes.
PROGRAM-MING LANGUAGE	Digital computers only understand binary code. This is very difficult to write and read it back for checking (it would consist of vast lists of 1s and 0s). To simplify the matter, languages were developed to allow "English"-like commands to be used that are subsequently automatically converted into binary code.
PROMPT	A message displayed on the monitor screen which asks you to perform some action (e.g. enter a data item) and shows that the computer is ready to accept a command or instruction.
PSTN	Public Switched Telephone Network — the "normal" analogue service.
PSRO	Professional Standards Review Organisation
QWERTY	Refers to the first six top left-hand letters of a typewriter-style keyboard. Most keyboards are QWERTY, although some special keyboard layouts are in limited usage.
RAM	Random Access Memory. The memory present in the computer that is used by programs and data when the computer is switched on. Computer instructions and data to be manipulated are held in RAM for ease of speed of access and processing. Generally speaking, the greater the RAM the better. Any data held in RAM is lost if the system is switched off or reset.

READ CODES — A coding system for medical terms, designed to be used by clinicians and to provide a means of recording all significant elements of a care encounter.

RECORD — In a data file, a group of data fields that collectively represent information about a single entity.

REDIRECTION — Routing of the output generated by a computer command to a destination other than its standard or default destination (e.g. sending a listing of files which would normally be displayed on screen, to the printer instead).

REMOTE ACCESS — Access to a system or to information therein, typically by telephone or communications network, by a user who is physically removed from the system.

REMOVABLE MEDIA — Floppy disks and tape cartridges are called removable media because they can be removed from the computer. Removable hard disks can also be obtained.

RESET — The computer is returned to the state it was prior to booting the system. Any data in RAM is lost.

RISC — Reduced Instruction Set Computer — a computer whose CPU has a limited set of commands it can execute, but which it does very fast. (See also CISC).

ROM — Read Only Memory. Memory which is built into the machine and is permanent (i.e not lost when the power is switched off). Provides a means to boot a computer when initially switched on.

ROOT DIRECTORY — The main or top directory in a computer filestore.

RS232 — The commonest form of serial interface, having 25 pins.

SCAMC — Symposium on Computer Applications in Medical Care — an annual meeting held in Washington USA in November.

SCREEN — The part of the monitor which displays text and images produced by the program.

SEMANTICS   Meaning of symbols and codes.

SERIAL PORT   A means of transmitting data. Each byte is broken down into bits and each is transmitted sequentially down a single wire. The speed is slower than parallel, but the distance over which transmission can take place is increased.

SERVER   (See FILESERVER).

SGML   Standard Generalised Markup Language — a standard approach to representing text including layout, pitch and fonts, which can be used to exchange documents without loss of any features.

SHELL   Part of the operating system which interacts with the user and interprets user commands for the computer to execute. Shell commands are unique to a particular shell. Shell scripts are programs written using shell commands.

SNOMED   Systematised Nomenclature of Medicine — a multi-axial classification system for medicine.

SOFTWARE   Collective term for computer programs and data files.

SPECIFI-CATION   A detailed description of the designs, actions and physical resources which are needed to meet a set of requirements.

SPOOLER   A program which places tasks (typically printing tasks) into a queue. As a job is sent to the printer it is placed in a queue until the printer is available.

SQL   Structured Query Language — a standardised approach to writing a database enquiry which can be understood by any SQL compliant database.

STANDARD   A specification established by consensus and approved by a recognised body, that provides, for common and repeated use, rules, guidelines or characteristics for activities or their results. Standards are essential where there is to be any meaningful exchange of data between systems.

STANDARD INPUT	The keyboard — the default device normally used to enter data or commands into the computer.
STANDARD OUTPUT	The screen — the default device normally used for data output.
SYNONYM	Two terms designating the same concept or entity.
SYNTAX	Rules for the structuring of words into sentences, or computer commands, or electronic messages.
SYSTEM	The combination of hardware and software which processes information for you.
SYSTEM DISK	Same as Bootable Disk.
SYSTEM FILES	Files that relate to the operating system and/or set-up of the computer, typically used in respect of these few files required for booting.
SYSTEMS ANALYSIS	The process of assessing whether a particular task is suitable for computerisation and the type of hardware and software required to do it.
TAPE STREAMER	A magnetic tape device like a cassette recorder. Tape streamers are widely used to make backup copies of a system's information, held on hard disk, in a matter of minutes. The alternative is to use a large number of floppy disks, changing them as each one fills.
TCP/IP	Transport Control Program/Internet Protocol — a communications protocol, very widely used but not conforming to standards.
TERM	Word or phrase used to designate a concept.
TERMINAL	Usually a keyboard and screen connected to a central computer and its CPU.
TERMINAL EMULATION	See EMULATION.
THESAURUS	A thesaurus is a tool which links together words with similar meanings.
TRANSACTION	Any instruction from a user and executed by a computer.

TP   Transaction Processing — an operational system which performs transactions.

TURNKEY   A computer system that is purchased from a vendor and that can be installed and operated with minimal modification.
SYSTEM

UMLS   Unified Medical Language System — a meta-thesaurus project designed to provide a way of translating between medical classification systems.

UNIX   The operating system adopted by the open systems movement as the basic operating environment for machines from workstation/large PC size up to mainframe systems.

UNTDED   United Nations Trade Data Elements Directory — the directory of data elements for use in EDIFACT messages.

USER   A term used to indictate the ease with which a program can be used by people with little or no computing experience.
FRIENDLY

USER ID   The name by which a user is known to a computer system. Usually coupled with a password.

USER   Method of interaction between users and information systems. This includes graphical user interface (GUI), dialogue model, particular devices and general ergonomy features.
INTERFACE

VDU   Visual Display Unit — A device (e.g. television screen) for viewing output from the computer. VDU screens are often limited to displaying 24 lines of text with up to 80 characters per line, although this can be modified through the use of presentation managers (e.g. Windows).

WAN   Wide Area Network

WE/EB   Western Europe EDIFACT Board — the body responsible for ratifying EDI messages in Europe.

WILDCARD   A symbol that can be substituted for a class of characters. The asterisk symbol (*) is the most commonly used wildcard.

WHO — World Health Organisation — the international body responsible for betterment of population health.

WONCA — World Organisation of National Colleges, Academies and Academic Associations of General Practitioners/Family Physicians

WORD PROCESSING PROGRAM — A program which turns your computer into a machine for processing text. Text can be entered, edited, saved, recovered, copied and moved. Extra text can be added from a disk. Standard letters and forms can be prepared and personalised by use of the mail merge.

WORM — Write Once, Read Many (optical disk) device — a way of storing large amounts of data in an inerasable form.

WORKSTATION — A term used to mean a PC, node or terminal. It is a device that has local processing capabilities and is operated by a user.

WRITE PROTECT — A way of protecting data stored on a disk from alteration or erasure — similar to that used on audio cassettes to prevent overwriting.

X.25 — Communication protocol based on lower 4 layers only of OSI stack.

X.400 — Electronic mail exchange and message handling protocol OSI compliant.

X.500 — Directory services for wide area networks.

Useful addresses

BSI
British Standards Institution
2 Park Street
London W1A 2BS

Tel 071–629 9000
Fax 071–629 0506

CEN
Comite Europeen de Normalisation
Rue de Stassart 36
B-1050 Brussels
Belgium

Tel +32 2 511 7455
Fax +32 2 511 8723

CSA
Computing Services Association
Hanover House
73/74 High Holborn
London WC1V 6LE

Tel 071–405 2171
Fax 071–404 4119

DoH
Department of Health
NHS Information Systems Directorate
Market Towers
1 Nine Elms Lane
Vauxhall
London SW8 5NQ

Tel 071–720 2188
Fax 071–622 9514

EWOS
European Workshop for Open Systems
Rue de Stassart 36, 7th Floor
B-1050 Brussels
Belgium

Tel +32 2 511 7455
Fax +32 2 511 8723

HL7
Health Level Seven
P O Box 66111
Chicago
IL 6066666–9998
U S A

Tel +1 301 340 0016
Fax +1 708 616 9099

IEEE
Institute of Electrical and Electronic Engineers
345 East 47th Street
New York
NY 10017
U S A

ISO
International Standards Organisation
Rue de Varembe 1
Case Postale 56
CH-1211 Geneva 20
Switzerland

Tel +41 22 341 240
Fax +41 22 333 430

NHS CCC
Centre for Coding and Classification
Woodgate
Loughborough
Leicestershire LE11 2TG

Tel 0509 211411
Fax 0509 211611

NHS IMC
Information Management Centre
19 Calthorpe Road
Edgbaston
Birmingham B15 1RP

Tel 021–454 1112
Fax 021–455 9340

NLM
National Library of Medicine
8600 Rockville Pike
Bethesda, MA 20209
U S A

Tel +1 301 496 6921

SITPRO (EDIFACT Service)
Venture House
29 Glasshouse Street
London W1R 5RG

Tel 071–287 3525
Fax 071–287 5751

WE/EB
Western Europe EDIFACT Board
DG XIII-D/4
CEC, 200 Rue de la Loi
B-1040 Brussels
Belgium

Tel +32 2 235 3998

Index